CLEAN KETO LIFESTYLE

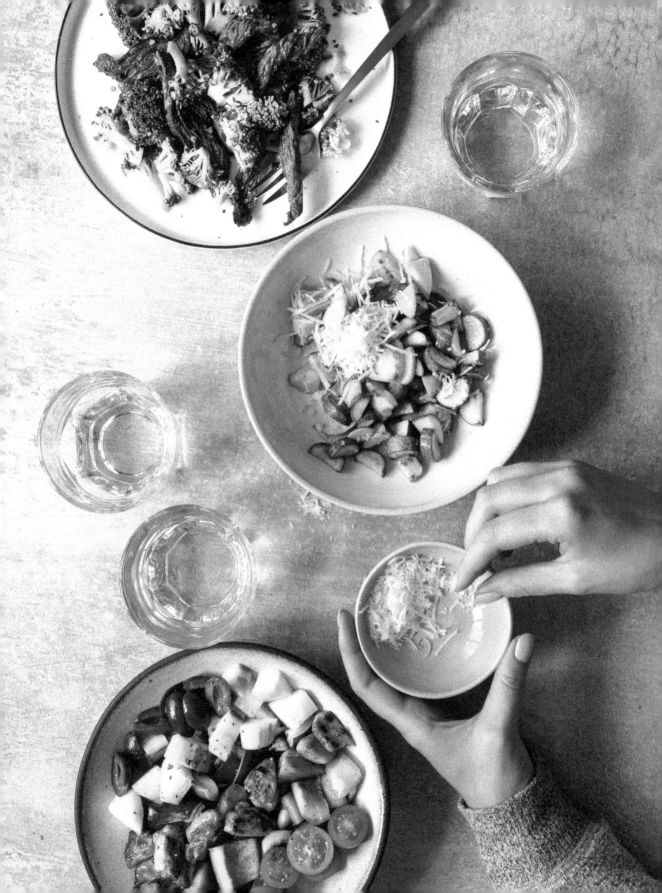

CLEAN KETO LIFESTYLE

The Complete Guide to
Transforming Your Life and Health

KARISSA LONG

ROCKRIDGE
PRESS

Cover Designer: Amy King and Merideth Harte
Interior Designer: Nami Kurita
Photo Art Director: Karen Beard
Editor: Pippa White
Production Editor: Andrew Yackira
Art Director: Amy King
Art Production Manager: Sue Bischofberger
Photography: © 2018 Nadine Greeff, cover and all interiors except p70; © 2018 Evi Abeler, p70.
Illustration: © 2018 Inspiring/Shutterstock p61, 62, 64, 65, 67, 68; graphix/Shutterstock p62, 63, 68; Charlie Layton p63, 66.

ISBN: Print 978-1-64152-325-7 | eBook 978-1-64152-326-4

TO MY HUSBAND, BRAD—
my best friend and biggest cheerleader. Thank you
for encouraging me to follow my passion.

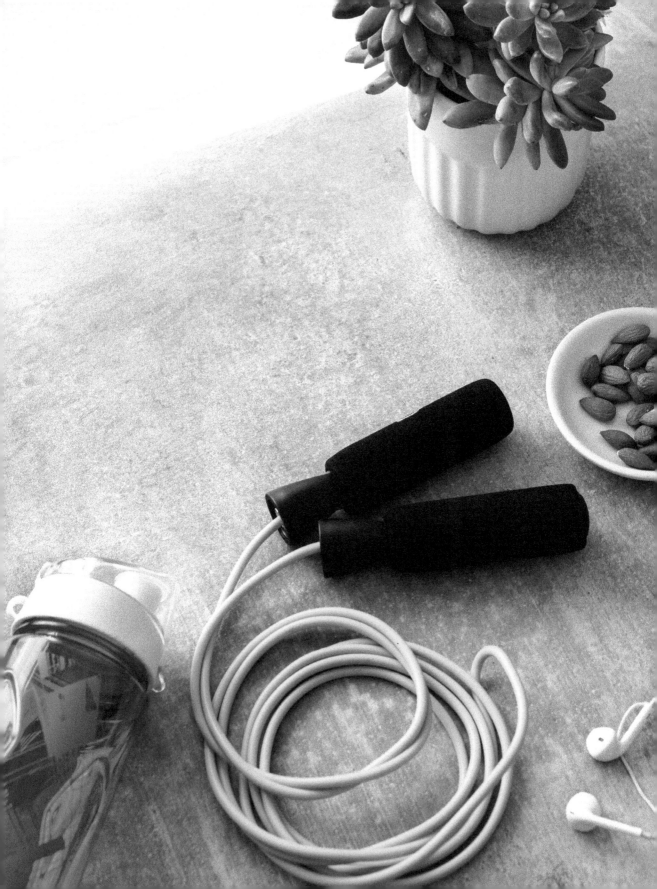

CONTENTS

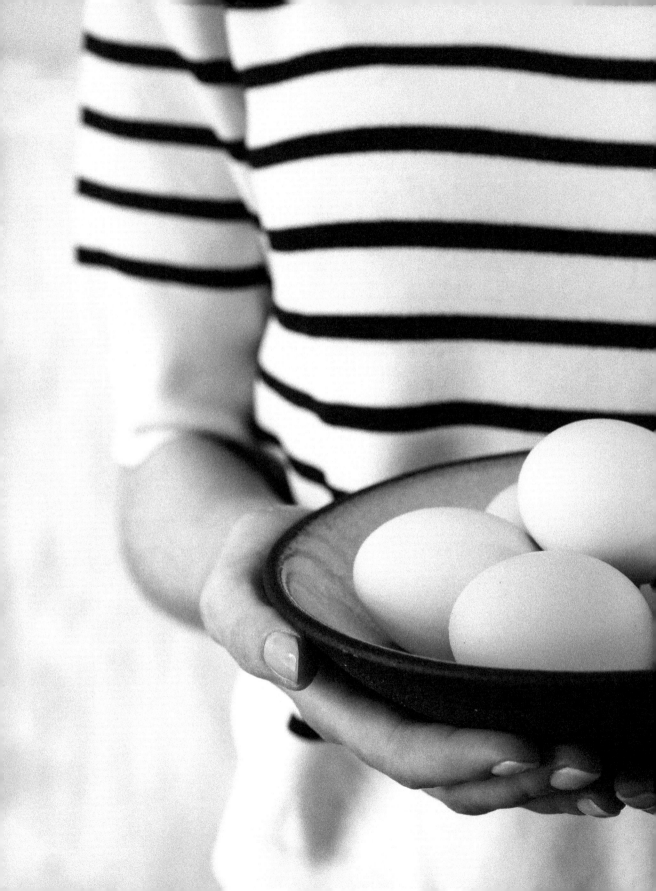

INTRODUCTION

As a Global Health Coach and Ketogenic Expert, my mission is to help everyone feel empowered to change their health for the better through a Clean Keto Lifestyle. This means doing the ketogenic diet the right way: free of processed foods with artificial ingredients and full of fresh, nutrient-dense fats, proteins, and vegetables.

I've spent over a decade transforming and fine-tuning my own health, as well as researching how what we put in our bodies and how we live our lives impacts our overall well-being. I found the ketogenic diet during my personal struggles with a debilitating autoimmune disease, and it completely transformed my life. Believe me when I say that it can transform yours, too! I went from a fast-food-eating, soda-pop-drinking sugar addict to a clean-eating, fat-burning machine!

Unfortunately, with the growing popularity of the ketogenic diet also comes a ton of misinformation, clever marketing by food companies, and improper implementation. As an Integrated Nutrition Health Coach, I am on a mission to change people's perspectives on what the ketogenic diet really is. It is *not* all about meat and cheese! It is actually far from that, and within this book I am going to share the knowledge I've gained through my personal wellness journey and comprehensive training to show you how to thrive on the ketogenic diet.

What makes a Clean Keto Lifestyle so different from all the other diets or wellness programs out there is that it is focused on improving your health first and foremost. My program also strips out all of the unnecessary steps that other keto gurus insist upon, like tediously tracking macros, restricting calories, and weighing your food. In my opinion, these steps make a keto lifestyle hard, and my goal is to make it *easy*, and thus sustainable. As you follow my program, your body will heal itself, excess weight will melt off, your energy levels will skyrocket, and you'll start to feel amazing.

My Story

For the first 25 years of my life, I admittedly neglected my health. Like many Americans, I survived by consuming what was easy and close by. I drank way too much diet soda and coffee. I ate prepackaged granola bars, thinking they were a healthy snack. I ate lots of fast food and ordered takeout frequently. I was always trying out the latest diets, hoping that I could crack the code and finally lose weight. Every diet I tried, though, would only last a few days before I reverted back to my old habits. It was extremely frustrating, not only because I couldn't stick with any diet, but also because I was always tired, carried excess weight, and felt like I was living in a mental fog.

Then, one day my body said enough is enough. I was diagnosed with a debilitating autoimmune disease called ulcerative colitis. I was told at the time that the only way to manage this disease was to take prescription drugs, and I followed those orders for years but still experienced flare-ups of awful symptoms. I was constantly worried that I was going to need surgery to remove a section of my colon, and I was in a very dark place. The most frustrating part was that my doctor could not explain what was causing my issues. I felt helpless and scared.

That is when I finally got serious about my health. I decided to take my health into my own hands. I read tons of medical books, attended nutrition seminars, and pored over scientific research studies. I concluded that the root cause of my disease was my diet. As a last-ditch effort, I slowly transitioned to a grain-free diet, and remarkably, my symptoms began to improve. I would still have flare-ups, but they were less frequent.

Then, one day I stumbled across a medical research paper that introduced me to the idea of the ketogenic diet, and that is when my life changed forever. My initial reaction was, *So you are telling me that I should eat 75 percent fat on this diet?!* I couldn't wrap my brain around it, but the more research I did, the more I realized that this was real, and that all of the science made perfect sense. I began implementing the ketogenic diet immediately, and never looked back.

Within a few months, I had shed the excess weight, I had more energy, my focus improved, I slept better, my skin got clearer, my cravings dramatically decreased, and to my surprise, my autoimmune disease went into remission! Even more astonishing was the fact that I didn't once feel like I was on a "diet." I was eating delicious and satisfying foods (including bacon!), and never felt like I was depriving myself. In fact, I felt balanced and content—better than I had ever felt in my life. I was thriving, and it was then that I realized the ketogenic diet is so much more than just a diet; it is a sustainable and incredible way of living that has implications far beyond just losing weight.

The improvement in my quality of life created a passion in me to help others do the same. I launched a company, Clean Keto Lifestyle, devoted to helping people transition into a sustainable keto lifestyle so they can feel better and thrive. I love the work I do, and I'm proud to say that since starting my company, I've helped thousands of people achieve their health goals with a ketogenic way of life. And there are so many more people I want to reach!

What I have found with all of my clients is that they are looking for a true lifestyle change—not just a quick fix. They want to be set up for success and given an all-encompassing plan to follow that will ensure they get results that are sustainable for life.

So, I wrote this book to show each and every person how to put a keto lifestyle into practice. In the following chapters, I'll provide you with a blueprint for creating your very own Clean Keto Lifestyle. I'll explain the science behind the ketogenic diet, what steps you should take to prepare, provide five weeks of meal plans, give you my go-to exercises, share over 75 delicious and nutritious keto recipes, and finally, I'll supply you with tips to incorporate keto into your life for good—even in social situations where it seems like eating keto may be challenging.

Let's get started—ready, set, ketosis!

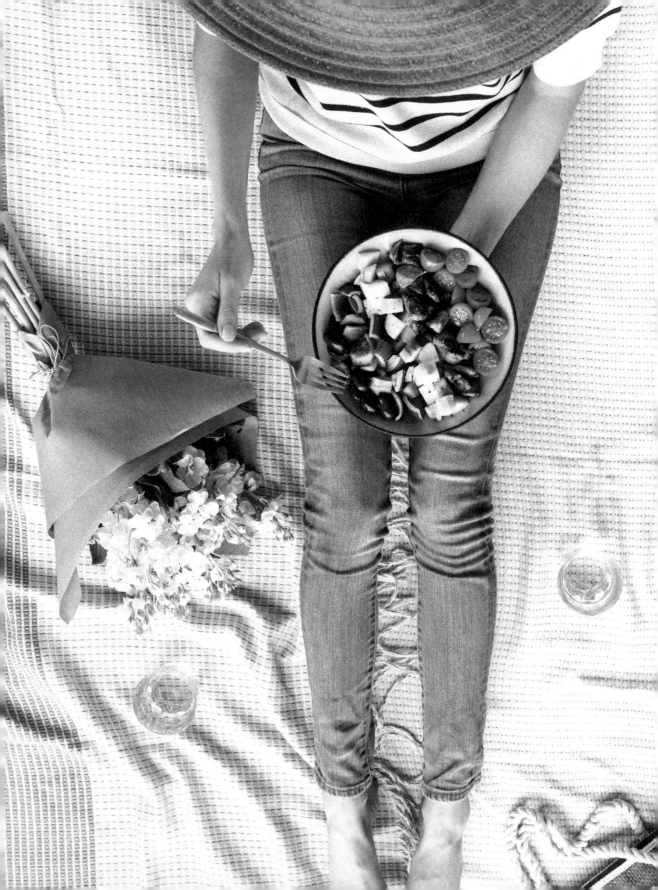

PART ONE
Clean Keto Living

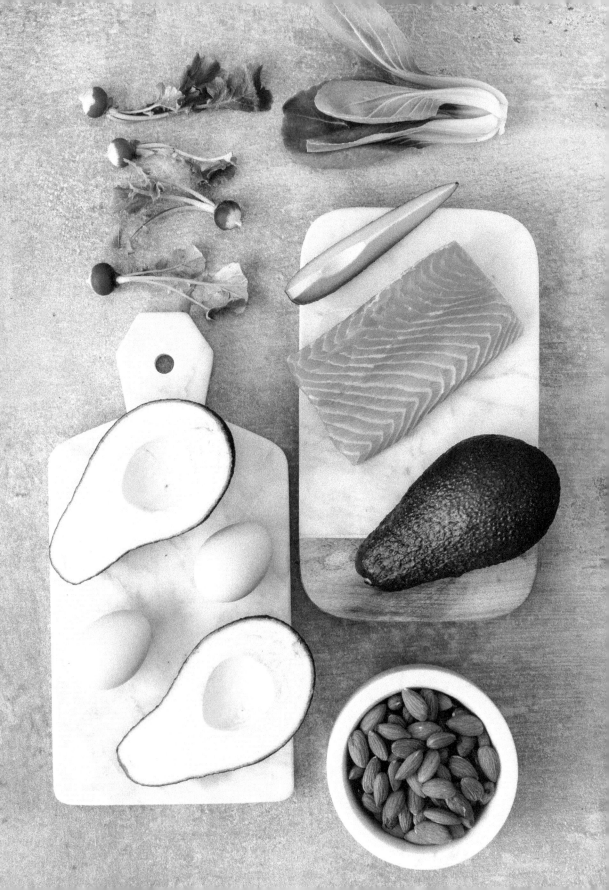

1

THE KETO WAY

Mastering and living a Clean Keto Lifestyle can be easy, convenient, and delicious, but it does require knowing some basics, including how and why the diet works, what the benefits are, and the best ways to make it a lasting lifestyle.

Don't worry—I've got you covered. This chapter is going to break it all down so you can start putting it into practice immediately.

I have been helping clients master the ketogenic diet for a long time now, and what I have found is that knowledge *truly* is power. If you are informed, you are empowered to make good decisions. If you know what certain foods do to your body, then you can choose wisely and feel confident in your choices.

So, whether you are a keto newbie or have some experience with keto, I urge you to soak up all the information in the following pages so you can set yourself up for lasting success.

How the Ketogenic Diet Works

Did you know that your body has two fuel sources?

The first one is **glucose**. Glucose is created by your body from the carbohydrates that you eat in grains, breads, pastas, sugar, and starches, to name a few. Glucose is a readily available fuel source for your body to use for energy, but it is not long-lasting, and the process of converting carbs to glucose sends your blood sugar on a roller-coaster ride that I like to call the "glu-coaster."

Here is how it works:

1. After you consume carbohydrates (think refined grains and sugars), your body begins to digest them into glucose.
2. This process of converting carbs to glucose causes a spike in your blood sugar and gives you a temporary energy boost (this is where the term "sugar high" comes from).
3. In response to this aggressive blood sugar spike (and because a glucose overdose in your bloodstream can be toxic), your body reacts by signaling to the pancreas to release the hormone insulin, which acts to remove the excess glucose from your bloodstream.
4. The released insulin works swiftly to transport the glucose out of your bloodstream to burn as fuel and then puts the rest in storage (more on this in a minute).
5. As the insulin removes the glucose from your bloodstream, your blood sugar subsequently drops, your energy level declines, and you feel hungry again.
6. So you eat more carbs, and the cycle begins again . . .

This process is why most people get an afternoon energy crash around 3:00 p.m. and start craving sweets or candy. One piece of comfort I can give you is that it is not your lack of willpower that causes these cravings. It is your body saying, "Hey! My blood sugar is low, and I need more energy—give me carbs now!"

If being on the never-ending "glu-coaster" wasn't bad enough, I have one more important fact for you. Depending on how much energy you need (which is based primarily on your physical activity level), you burn that specific amount of glucose and the rest is stored in your body. Some of the excess glucose is converted into glycogen and stored in your liver and muscle tissues for future use. But the remaining glucose that your body didn't use is stored as FAT in the form of triglycerides. That's right, your body stores the excess glucose in your fat cells and essentially forgets about it.

Then, of course, the whole cycle starts again. You eat more carbs at your next meal, you jump on the "glu-coaster," your body uses what it needs for energy and stores the rest as fat. And those fat cells keep piling up. *This* is the reason you gain weight.

But I have good news! Your body has another fuel source called **ketones**.

Ketones are these incredible little energy pods created by your body from stored fat. Yes, you heard me correctly: You can turn those stored fat cells into energy. And not just any kind of energy—energy that is long lasting and consistent, with no afternoon crashes. When you use ketones for energy, your body is using its own stored fat as fuel. Thus, you start losing weight. Brilliant, right?

The goal of the ketogenic diet is to capitalize on all of this by training your body to start burning ketones for energy instead of glucose. This phenomenon is called ketosis. When your body is in a state of ketosis, it becomes a literal fat-burning machine.

So to summarize, these are the basics:

What is a ketogenic diet? It is a low-carb, moderate-protein, high-fat diet designed to exhaust glucose levels and prompt the body to provide an alternative source of energy to the brain. These alternative energy sources are called ketones, which are produced by the liver using stored fat.

What is ketosis? When the body takes stored fat through the liver and produces ketones (small molecules used as fuel throughout the body), it is called ketosis.

Why do you want to be in ketosis? When you are in a state of ketosis, your body literally becomes a fat-burning machine! Ketosis is the way for humans to operate most efficiently and can lead to numerous benefits such as weight loss, increased energy, improved focus, better sleep, clear skin, strength gain, reduced appetite, better digestion, and balanced mood, to name a few.

Well, it's all about what you eat and how much you eat of each macronutrient (also known as "**macros**").

There are three types of macronutrients in the human diet: fats, proteins, and carbohydrates. On the ketogenic diet, your daily macronutrient breakdown should be as follows:

75% healthy fats

20% quality protein

5% carbohydrates

It's true—approximately 75 percent of what you eat each day will come from fat. Fat is actually the most essential macronutrient that the body needs. You need fat to live. It keeps you feeling full and satisfied, prevents cravings, and is 100 percent necessary for you to get into ketosis.

When following this macronutrient ratio, you can get into ketosis within two to seven days, depending on your current glycogen supply, body type, and activity level. This means you can start reaping the amazing benefits of ketosis in as little as one week!

The Benefits of a Keto Diet

There are several different motivators for starting the ketogenic diet. For many it is weight loss, while others are looking for more energy, clearer skin, or better mental focus. For me, the ketogenic diet eliminated my terrible ulcerative colitis symptoms.

Let's review the numerous benefits of the diet in detail.

FAT LOSS

By definition, being in a state of ketosis means you are burning stored fat for energy. With a Clean Keto Lifestyle, weight loss can often be significant and can happen quickly, because not only are you turning your body into a fat-burning machine, but you are also ridding your body of processed foods, artificial ingredients, and sugars that interfere with your appetite hormones.

When you are in ketosis, you seldom feel hungry, your cravings subside, and you don't have to worry about counting calories. No more food drama.

IMPROVED BRAIN FUNCTION

Other than fat loss, another big reason so many people turn to the ketogenic diet is for improved cognitive function, mental clarity, and to *finally* lift that brain fog once and for all. In fact, a sharper mind is most likely one of the first benefits you will notice when achieving ketosis.

This is because, in comparison to glucose, ketones are actually an upgraded fuel source for your brain. Studies have shown that ketones can provide as much as 70 percent of the brain's energy needs and are more energy efficient than glucose.

FAST AND SUSTAINABLE ENERGY

One of the most profound benefits of the ketogenic diet is wonderful, long-lasting energy! On a ketogenic diet, your energy levels are stable throughout the day, meaning no midafternoon slumps, no insatiable cravings for sugar, and no need for caffeine pick-me-ups. This is because when you get off the "glu-coaster," your blood sugar levels are stabilized.

Most of my clients experience an increase in general energy levels within the first few weeks. Once again, this phenomenon is the result of your body being fueled more efficiently by ketones.

DECREASED INFLAMMATION

Inflammation is always present in our bodies. Some is advantageous, like when you get a scrape or a bruise and your body uses inflammation to heal. However, chronic inflammation can become a problem.

A huge benefit of being in ketosis is that it can lower inflammation, because free radical production (which is extremely inflammatory) is reduced when you're burning ketones for energy.

Also, when you remove processed foods from your diet, you consequently eliminate all inflammation-producing additives, artificial ingredients, preservatives, and sweeteners, and instead fill your plate with real foods full of minerals and vitamins that work to decrease internal inflammation in your body.

OTHER BENEFITS

My clients have also reported better sleep, less acne, better muscle tone, and a balanced mood after implementing the ketogenic diet, which makes them look and feel younger!

Research also links the ketogenic diet to a multitude of other benefits, including cancer treatment/prevention, improving chronic disease and autoimmune disorders, Alzheimer's treatment, neuroprotection, and brain trauma injury healing.

Foods to Eat and Avoid on Keto

HEALTHY FATS

- Animal Fats
  + Butter
  + Ghee
  + Lard
  + Mayonnaise
  + Tallow
- Nut Butters
  + Almond butter
  + Cocoa butter
  + Coconut butter

- Unrefined Oils
  + Avocado oil
  + Coconut oil
  + Extra-virgin olive oil
  + Macadamia oil
  + MCT oil

- Other
  + Avocado
  + Coconut milk, full-fat
  + Nuts (almonds, pecans, macadamia nuts, walnuts)
  + Olives

QUALITY PROTEIN

- Eggs
- Beef
  + Ground
  + Tenderloin
- Chicken
  + Ground
  + Quarters
  + Thighs
  + Whole
- Organ Meats
  + Collagen powder
  + Liver

  + Tripe
- Pork
  + Bacon
  + Chops
  + Ground
  + Sausage
  + Tenderloin
- Seafood
  + Salmon
  + Sardines
  + Scallops
  + Sea bass
  + Shrimp

  + Trout
  + Tuna
- Steak
  + Filet
  + Flank
  + Rib-eye
  + Skirt
- Turkey
  + Ground
  + Quarters
  + Slices, precooked
  + Thighs
  + Whole

NONSTARCHY VEGETABLES

- Artichokes
- Asparagus
- Bok choy
- Broccoli
- Brussels sprouts
- Cabbage
- Cauliflower
- Celery
- Chard
- Chives
- Cucumber
- Eggplant
- Endive
- Fennel
- Garlic
- Green beans
- Kale
- Leeks
- Lettuce
- Mushrooms
- Okra
- Onions
- Peppers
- Radicchio
- Radishes
- Rhubarb
- Spinach
- Sprouts
- Tomatoes
- Water chestnuts
- Zucchini

BEVERAGES

- Bone broth
- Coffee (no sweetener)
- Seltzer/sparkling water, unflavored
- Tea (unsweetened and not instant)
- Water

FLAVORINGS

- Black pepper, ground
- Dried herbs and spices
- Fresh herbs (basil, cilantro, mint, oregano, parsley, rosemary, thyme, etc.)
- Lemon
- Lime
- Mustard (yellow, Dijon)
- Pink Himalayan salt
- Vinegars (apple cider, balsamic, and red wine)

FOODS TO EAT IN MODERATION

- Dairy
  (1 cup max per day)
  + **Cheese, full-fat**
  + **Cream, heavy**
  + **Greek yogurt, full-fat, plain**

- Fruits
  (½ cup max per day)
  + **Blackberries**
  + **Blueberries**
  + **Raspberries**
  + **Strawberries**

FOODS TO AVOID

- Most fruits—apples, bananas, oranges, etc. (Fruit contains sugar in the form of fructose, which can only be processed in the body by your liver. When the liver gets overloaded with fructose, it stores the excess as fat.)

- Starchy vegetables (potatoes, sweet potatoes, plantains, butternut squash, etc.)

- All grains and starches (bread, wheat, corn, rice, cereal, etc.)

- Beer, ciders, and sweet wines/liquors

- Refined oils (vegetable, grapeseed, canola, soybean, corn)

- Margarine

- Sugar of all kinds (white and brown sugar, powdered sugar, honey, maple syrup, agave, high-fructose corn syrup, evaporated cane juice, etc.)

- Artificial sweeteners (Splenda, Sweet'n Low, Equal, Truvia, etc.)

- Processed foods

- Soda/diet soda

- Fruit juice

- Fruit-based smoothies

- Energy drinks

- Low-fat and diet products containing artificial ingredients/sweeteners

Beyond a Diet: Clean Keto Lifestyle

My mantra at Clean Keto Lifestyle is "Be your best self." I want each person to adopt a healthy way of living—not just in the short term, but for the rest of their lives.

By following the principles of a Clean Keto Lifestyle, you are reprogramming your body and upgrading its fuel source. You are healing and getting your body back to the way it was intended to function. When we live in harmony with our bodies, everything is easier. No more fighting cravings or starving ourselves. No more food drama.

This is what makes my plan sustainable. It is about providing our bodies with nourishment. It is about eating real foods that our bodies recognize and can digest easily. And it is about treating our bodies with respect and care.

My clients lose weight and are able to keep it off because they do it the right way, without starvation, diet pills, or excessive exercise. When you rid your body of all forms of sugar, inflammatory grains, artificial ingredients, and processed foods, while at the same time embracing healthy fats, quality protein, and a wide range of nutrient-dense vegetables, you open up a whole new way of living. And I am so excited for you to experience this new lifestyle!

KETO IN THE REAL WORLD

Most keto books focus solely on recipes—which are great—but they are only one facet of living keto. This book provides you with the tools you need to create healthy habits that last a lifetime, such as grocery shopping strategies, advice on how to stay keto in social situations, and specific techniques for dining out.

That is why this book is called *Clean Keto Lifestyle* (emphasis on the lifestyle!). It doesn't help to only be keto in your own kitchen—my clients tell me they want help staying keto when they are out in the world, living their lives. I'm here to tell you that you don't have to choose between being a social person and being keto. You can have it all!

My hope is that you can soak up the information in this book and put it into practice to set yourself up for a successful new lifestyle. Take keto out of the kitchen and live your life with freedom, confident that you are able to make choices that keep you on track!

Making the Keto Lifestyle Easy

Are you ready to make some permanent lifestyle changes? I am here to help you get off the "glu-coaster" once and for all, and start living your life on the smooth and steady ketone highway. Picture this:

- You know exactly what to eat to ensure you are following the ketogenic diet principles correctly without the need for tedious macro-tracking and calorie counting.

- You are eating healthy, satisfying meals that are full of nutrients that nourish and heal your body.

- You're "eating to live" instead of "living to eat," because you finally have food freedom and no longer have insatiable cravings.

All of this is possible, and in the following pages, I will give you the blueprint to achieving amazing results with no second-guessing or frustrating learning curve.

First, we are going to start with preparation. Preparation is the key to success, and in the next chapter, I will guide you through planning macros, mastering meal prep, shopping for food, and setting up your kitchen.

Next, we will go over eating schedules and how to incorporate intermittent fasting into your daily life to maximize your results.

Once we are all organized, I'll provide you with five weeks of meal plans designed to get you into ketosis. Then, we will talk about how exercise fits into a Clean Keto Lifestyle, and I'll give you details on the best workouts to complement a ketogenic diet. After that, I'll share my foolproof tips and tricks for navigating social situations so you'll be ready for keto in the real world!

The second part of this book is dedicated to keto recipes, and I've included over 75 to make it all easy and delicious.

By the end of this book, you'll have all the tools you need to take control of your health, to free yourself from diets for good, to overcome those traps that have been keeping you stuck, and to ultimately master a Clean Keto Lifestyle.

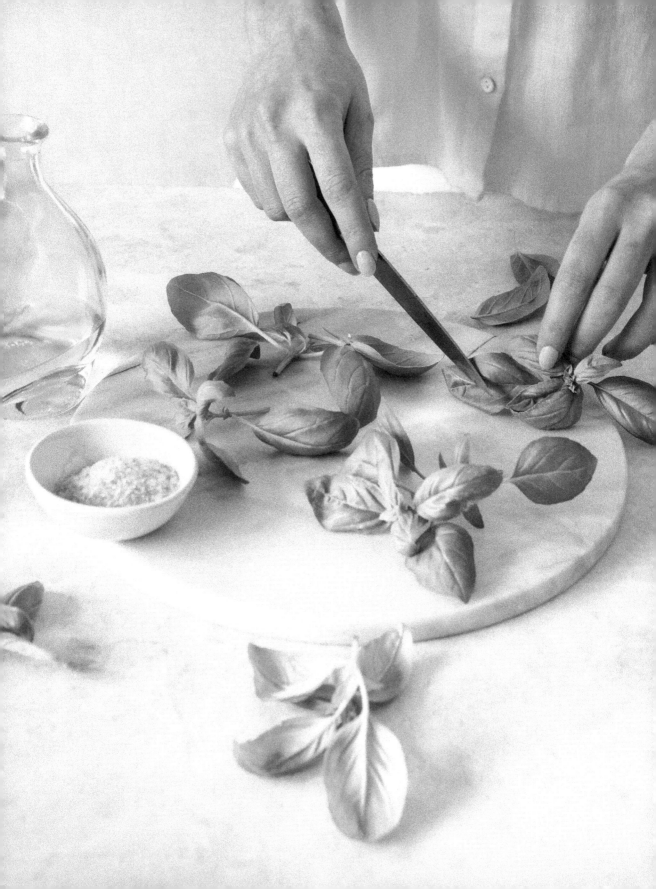

2

MEAL PREP &
THE KETO KITCHEN

Before we jump into the meal plans, we need to get organized. I sincerely believe that preparation equals success. The purpose of this chapter is to get you ready for a Clean Keto Lifestyle, so it's essential to read and follow these steps.

Planning Your Macros

A Clean Keto Lifestyle is rooted in the principles of real, whole foods. Yes, you can lose weight on the ketogenic diet by eating low-carb processed foods, consuming refined oils, and eating factory-farmed meat. But the key to optimal health is eliminating food toxins like chemical additives, sugar, omega-6 seed oils, trans fats, grains, and starches that lead to chronic inflammation in the body. Instead, your diet will center around foods that encourage healing and weight loss. These foods are healthy unrefined fats, grass-fed meats, pastured poultry, wild-caught seafood, organic raw nuts/seeds, and farm-fresh nonstarchy vegetables.

The secret to getting into ketosis is ensuring that you eat the right combination of these food categories each day. As a reminder, the macronutrient ratio guidelines for the ketogenic diet are as follows:

75% healthy fats

20% quality protein

5% carbohydrates

These percentages are daily goals, so each individual meal doesn't need to follow these guidelines exactly. I do recommend that you have fat at each meal to keep you satiated. And to be clear, the carbohydrate portion of your diet should come from vegetables and berries—not grains or sugars.

In the Clean Keto Lifestyle approach, I don't believe tedious macro tracking is necessary. Instead, I teach my clients a different technique. I call it the **8-3-6 formula**. It focuses on serving sizes and how you build your daily meals. To follow this formula:

- Aim to eat **8** servings of fat each day—
1 SERVING = 1 tablespoon (the size of your thumb)

- Aim to eat **3** servings of protein each day —
1 SERVING = ⅓ or ¼ of a cup (the size of your palm)

- Aim to eat **6** servings of non-starchy vegetables each day—
1 SERVING = 1 cup (the size of your fist)

Tracking macros really comes down to personal preference. Most of my clients find that this way of calculating their macros eliminates all the hassle, which makes it easier to maintain. But some people find that meticulously counting macros works best for them. As a result, I have included macronutrient information for each recipe included in this book. Experiment with which option works best for you.

FALLING OUT OF KETOSIS

Life happens and no one is perfect, so more likely than not, you are occasionally going to fall out of ketosis. It is not the end of the world. The key is getting back into ketosis as soon as you can.

Here are some techniques to help you get back into ketosis quickly.

Fast: Try to not eat for at least 16 to 24 hours after falling out of ketosis.

Pump up your MCT intake: MCTs are medium-chain triglycerides, which can be found in coconut oil, grass-fed butter, or as a concentrated oil in your health food store. MCTs are a form of saturated fatty acids that can be quickly absorbed and converted into ketone bodies by your liver.

Get moving: Being physically active can help you get into ketosis. When you exercise, you can deplete your body of its glycogen stores and force it to produce ketones for fuel.

The bottom line: To make this a true lifestyle, always keep moving forward, and don't let one slipup stop your progress. Be patient, don't be too hard on yourself, and keep your focus on the long term.

Setting Yourself Up for Success

Meal prep is a critical step toward achieving success. By planning and prepping your meals ahead of time, you have a strategy. No more impulsive, craving-driven decisions, no more long cook times, and no more excuses. All the chopping, roasting, and other prep work will already have been done, so all you'll need to do at mealtime is just assemble and eat.

Of course, it might sound intimidating to prep a whole week's worth of meals, but don't stress. I've included my foolproof tips to make it easier than you'd think.

START SIMPLE

The first trick of meal prepping is to avoid making it overly complicated. For the first few weeks, keep your meals simple. Forget the fat bombs, keto bread, and complicated recipes.

Instead, try eggs and bacon at breakfast, a roasted chicken salad with extra-virgin olive oil and vinegar dressing at lunch, and baked salmon with asparagus sautéed in coconut oil at dinner. The simpler your meals are, the easier and faster your prep work will be.

Starting with simple meals that are easy to put together will give you good practice and build your confidence.

COOKING IN BULK

Batch cooking is the most efficient way to use your time in the kitchen. Carve out a few hours on the weekend or after you get home from the grocery store to get organized. The goal of batch cooking is to have all of the time-consuming foods cooked or prepped ahead of time so you are just reheating and assembling throughout the week. First, prep your grocery haul. Here is the breakdown.

Proteins: Roast, bake, or poach your meats (chicken, beef, turkey, etc.) and seafoods (salmon, shrimp, tuna, etc.).

Vegetables: Wash and chop your veggies for salads. Roast or steam vegetables in a large batch, making sure to include lots of healthy fats.

Add-ons: Make sauces and dressings to use throughout the week.

Next, store your prepared food items in clear, sealed containers so you can locate them easily in the refrigerator. I recommend glass containers or BPA-free plastic.

If you plan to bring meals to work with you, assemble them ahead of time. Pack up a roasted protein with some veggies, build a salad and keep the dressing on the side, or blend up a keto-friendly smoothie and store it in the refrigerator.

MEAL PREP 101

When to Prep

Everyone's schedule is different, so figure out a time to prep meals that works for you. For the most part, you will need to carve out about two hours to get all your meal prepping done. Sunday is very popular with my clients, but if Wednesday night is when you have the most free time, by all means, do it then. The key is making meal prep a part of your lifestyle and fitting it into your calendar. Like anything in life, the more you do it, the better you get at it and the easier it becomes.

Which Meals to Prep

What to prep really comes down to your preferences and how busy you are in the upcoming week. Some weeks you will have no free time at night, so you'll need to prep all of your meals ahead of time. Other weeks you may have time to whip up a few quick 30-minute dishes.

I teach my clients to estimate how much food they need to prep by using this formula to build keto meals:

- Start with 1 serving of protein (chicken, salmon, steak, etc.)
- Cook it in 1 to 2 servings of healthy fat (coconut oil, avocado oil, grass-fed butter, ghee, lard)
- Add in at least 2 nonstarchy vegetables (greens, asparagus, broccoli, zucchini, cauliflower) that should be cooked or topped with 1 to 2 additional servings of healthy fat (extra-virgin olive oil, grass-fed butter)

Voilà! You have a Clean Keto Lifestyle–approved meal.

I tell my clients to write down how many meals they will need to have prepared ahead of time for the upcoming week. Then, based on the keto meal formula above, they can figure out how much to cook ahead of time.

For example, if you need five meals ready ahead of time, you would need to cook five servings of a protein and 10 servings of nonstarchy vegetables.

USING LEFTOVERS

Leverage your leftovers! When meal prepping, look for ways to use the same ingredients in your meals throughout the week, or simply have the same meal more than once a week by cooking double or triple batches. This way, you'll have fewer ingredients to buy and can meal prep even more efficiently.

For example, you can roast several chicken thighs at the beginning of the week for use in a delicious cobb salad for Monday's lunch, then serve the rest with roasted broccoli for a yummy dinner on another day.

To some people, leftovers can be boring. Feel free to liven up your leftover meal by doing the following:

- Add some toppings (nuts, seeds, a drizzle of oil, or fresh herbs).

- Serve it in a different manner (cold vs. warm, in a bowl vs. on a plate). These little changes can trick your brain into thinking it is a new dish.

- When in doubt, add hot sauce! Hot sauce livens up any dish it touches and is so versatile. Just make sure there are not any added sugars or other non-keto ingredients in the brand you choose.

THE KETO SHOPPING CART

Eating quality, wholesome food is the secret behind the success of a Clean Keto Lifestyle. In order to eat quality foods, you first need to buy them. Let's break down your keto shopping strategy.

Where to Shop . . . and How

Lucky for all of us, times are changing, and finding foods that are farm fresh, organic, and high quality is not only getting easier, but is also more affordable.

Here are a few shopping strategies that you can implement to ensure you get the best food for the lowest price.

GROCERY STORES

Shop the perimeter. Fresh foods found in the produce area, meat and seafood counter, dairy and egg section, and bulk bins normally are located around the edges of the store. These are the types of foods that you want to purchase.

Avoid the box. Look for foods that don't come in a box (most processed foods are packaged), and instead choose real foods that don't have an ingredient list because they are just one ingredient.

Read the labels.
- If you are buying something in a package, check that there are no added sugars or artificial ingredients. You should be able to recognize every ingredient on the label.
- Check the net carb count (total carbs minus fiber). Avoid anything that has a high net carb count per serving size. My rule of thumb is to choose foods with 5 grams of net carbs or less per serving size. Also, avoid anything that has more than 0 grams of "Added Sugars" on the label.
- Look for quality indicators, and opt for these foods:
  + Vegetables: local, non-GMO, and organic
  + Proteins: grass-fed, grass-finished, pastured, wild-caught
  + Fats, seeds, and nuts: organic, unrefined, non-GMO, raw

Buy in bulk. Take advantage of better pricing and/or sales.
- Compare prices. Always look at the price per unit for an item. For instance, an 8-ounce bag of almonds could be $7.99 on the shelf (approximately $1.00 per ounce), but in the bulk bin the price per ounce could be only $0.50.
- Stock up. If there is a great sale price on meats and seafood, by all means buy multiple quantities. You can always store the extra supply in your freezer and use it at a later time.

FARMERS' MARKETS

Freshest and healthiest. You can't beat the taste and nutrient-density of food that comes straight from a nearby farm. If possible, seek out farmers who use organic farming techniques.

Make friends with the farmer. Search online for local farmers' markets, and get to know the farmers. They will be your best allies when it comes to finding quality foods. Ask them questions about their farming methods, the freshest items they have in stock, and bulk pricing discounts.

Good value vs. quality. I find that the prices at farmers' markets are comparable to grocery stores, and the quality is far superior. Plus, you are supporting locally owned businesses, so it is a win-win.

Saves time. Shopping online is a great option for busy people who don't have time to go to the store each week and love the convenience of getting food shipped directly to their front door.

Hard-to-find foods. Depending on where you live, you may not have the ability to find quality foods at your local grocery store or farmers' market. If that is the case, purchasing foods online is a great option.

My favorites:
- Amazon
- Butcher Box
- Sizzlefish
- Thrive Market
- US Wellness Meats
- Vitacost

My personal shopping strategy is to buy pantry staples and healthy fats online for the best prices I can find, and then head to the farmers' market each week for fresh, in-season vegetables and proteins. Take some time to figure out the right strategy for you and where you live. The good news is that quality food is available to all of us now, so it really comes down to preference as to where you buy it.

Here are the keto brands that pass my high-quality standards.

PROTEINS

- Butcher Box (frozen grass-fed beef, heritage breed pork, and free-range chicken)
- Epic (dried meats and jerky)
- Safe Catch (canned tuna and other seafood)
- Sizzlefish (frozen wild-caught seafood)
- Vital Proteins (collagen and protein powders)
- Wild Planet (canned chicken, canned tuna, and other seafood)

HEALTHY FATS

- Artisana Organics (nut butters, coconut oil)
- Divina (olives)
- Fourth & Heart (ghee)
- Kerrygold (grass-fed butter)
- Manitoba Harvest (hemp hearts)
- Native Forest (full-fat coconut milk)
- NOW Foods (raw nuts, MCT oil)
- Nutiva (coconut oil)
- Primal Kitchen (mayo, avocado oil)
- Three Trees (almond milk)
- Thrive Market (raw nuts, ghee, nut butters, extra-virgin olive oil)

VEGETABLES

- Cascadian Organic Farm (frozen)
- Organic Girl Greens (refrigerated)
- Woodstock Organic (frozen)

CONDIMENTS AND SAUCES

- Annie's Organics (mustard)
- Coconut Secret (coconut aminos)
- Kettle & Fire (bone broth)
- Primal Kitchen (salad dressings and marinades)
- Rao's (tomato sauce)
- Red Boat (fish sauce)

Eating real foods that are free of additives, chemicals, and fillers not only aids in weight loss, but also improves your overall health. All of my clients agree with this philosophy, but the biggest pushback that I get is the **cost** of eating healthy.

I challenge you to take a different perspective and think about the following:

- **It's not that much more expensive.** According to weekly Agriculture Marketing Service reports distributed by the USDA, on average, organic vegetables are usually less than $1 more expensive per pound than their conventional counterparts. Do the math: If you are buying 2 pounds of produce, you are only paying $2 more for the organic version. When you look at the cost this way, it isn't that much higher.

- **Health is more important than shoes.** Why would you be cheap with what you are putting into your body? You only have one body, and it should be treated with respect. Most women I work with have no problem dropping $50 on an antiaging face cream or $200 on a shiny new pair of shoes, but cringe at spending $4.99 for a dozen delicious, vitamin-rich, pastured eggs. It really comes down to looking at the big picture and prioritizing how you spend your money.

- **Your health is an investment, not an expense.** It is worth a few extra dollars to eat the most nutrient-dense, vitamin-rich, flavorful foods out there. Have you ever noticed how luxury cars require "premium gas"? Yes, premium gas is a few cents more per gallon than the basic fuel at the gas station, but it optimizes the car's power and efficiency. The same goes for your body. Feed it premium food and get premium results!

The Keto Kitchen

Cooking at home instead of eating out when you first start the ketogenic diet allows you to be in control of what you are putting into your body. Restaurants can use refined oils and add sugars or other additives to their foods, which sets your progress back. Therefore, you ideally want to prepare your meals at home when you first begin the diet.

Don't worry if you are a "noncook." Having a well-stocked kitchen and the right equipment is essentially all you'll need to master keto cooking.

Here are the steps to create a Keto Kitchen:

STEP 1: CLEAN OUT YOUR KITCHEN

It sounds simple, but it's worth saying it in print: When you have bad food in the house, you'll eat it.

When first beginning the keto diet, it's a good idea to clean out your kitchen to remove any foods that no longer serve you (and may tempt you). I want you to set aside 30 minutes to go through your kitchen and toss or donate what you no longer will be eating. Remove any items that have the following ingredients or characteristics:

- Sugar or a sugar derivative listed as an ingredient
- Junk food or anything with highly processed ingredients
- Anything else on the "Foods to Avoid" list (see page 11)

Make sure to read the food labels on any packaged items. Condiments, sauces, and even pickles can have added sugars. Also, any ingredient you can't pronounce is a warning sign that it is not a real food, so get rid of it.

For some people, purging can be very liberating and motivating. If you are one of those people, this will be an easy task. Others find purging to be extremely hard because they think they are throwing away money and they have doubts about what they are actually going to eat. Be strong and push through these emotions. Think of this step as setting yourself up for success.

STEP 2: RESTOCK YOUR PANTRY AND REFRIGERATOR

Now that you have removed all the "fake foods" from your kitchen, let's replace them with the good stuff. Having a well-stocked kitchen with the following keto staples will ensure that you have the basics to whip up a keto meal at any time:

Keto Staples

FATS

- Avocado oil
- Coconut oil
- Extra-virgin olive oil
- Full-fat coconut milk
- Ghee/grass-fed butter
- Olives

CONDIMENTS

- Apple cider vinegar
- Balsamic vinegar (no sugar added)
- Coconut aminos
- Dijon mustard
- Mayonnaise (no sugar added)
- Red wine vinegar

DRIED SPICES

- Basil
- Black pepper
- Chili powder
- Cinnamon
- Cumin
- Garlic powder
- Onion powder
- Oregano
- Paprika
- Pink Himalayan salt
- Red pepper flakes
- Rosemary
- Thyme

REFRIGERATED ITEMS

- Bacon (no sugar added)
- Beef, ground (not lean)
- Cauliflower, whole head (can make into rice or cauli-mash)
- Cheese, full fat
- Chicken thighs
- Eggs
- Pickles/sauerkraut (to get your probiotics in)
- Salad greens (spinach, kale, arugula)
- Salmon fillets (or other fatty fish)
- Turkey, pre-cooked and sliced
- Vegetables, chopped (cucumber, broccoli, zucchini)

OTHER PERISHABLES

- Almonds
- Avocados
- Garlic bulbs
- Herbs, fresh (basil, mint, rosemary)
- Macadamia nuts
- Lemons
- Limes
- Onions
- Pecans
- Walnuts

PROTEINS

All of these should be packed in olive oil—preferably extra virgin olive oil, if possible.

- Canned anchovies
- Canned salmon
- Canned tuna

STEP 3: MAKE SURE YOU HAVE THE PROPER EQUIPMENT

Keto cooking doesn't require fancy equipment. But you do need a few basics. You most likely own a majority of these items already.

Kitchen Gadgets and Tools

MUST HAVES

- Baking sheet
- Blender
- Cheese grater
- Cutting board
- Food processor
- Mixing bowls
- Muffin tin
- Parchment paper/ aluminum foil
- Pot with a lid (large)
- Saucepan
- Sharp knife
- Skillets (1 small and 1 large)
- Storage containers (airtight, various sizes)
- Utensils (peeler, spatula, strainer)

NICE TO HAVES

- Cast iron skillet
- Slow cooker
- Spiralizer
- Steamer or steam basket
- Vitamix

Combining Keto with Intermittent Fasting

Another powerful way to set yourself up for success is to get into ketosis through intermittent fasting. If you don't eat for many hours, your body will naturally go into fat-burning mode. Intermittent fasting and ketosis paired together can be extremely effective.

WHAT IS FASTING?

Fasting is simply a type of eating schedule that is focused on giving your body an extended period of time between feedings. At any time of the day, your body is either in a fed or fasted state. When you are in a fed state, meaning your body is in the process of digesting food, you have higher insulin levels, so burning fat can be a challenge. When you are in a fasted state, which is usually 8 to 12 hours after your body has finished digesting food, your body is able to reach into your fat stores.

There are several intermittent fasting methods. Here are the most popular:

The 16/8 Method: Requires restricting your daily eating period to 8 hours and fasting for the remaining 16 hours

Eat-Stop-Eat: Requires fasting for 24 hours, 1 or 2 days per week

The 5:2 Diet: Requires eating only 500 to 600 calories on two nonconsecutive days during the week

HOW DOES IT WORK?

It makes perfect sense when you think about it. After you eat, your body spends the next few hours digesting that food, processing it, and burning what it can as fuel. Your body will take the most readily available energy source, which is the food you just ate, rather than the fat you have stored. This is especially true if you just consumed glucose (aka sugars and carbs), as your body prefers to burn glucose as energy before any other source.

If you are in a fasted state (you haven't recently consumed a meal), the body doesn't have that readily available glucose to use as energy, so it is more likely to pull from the fat stored in your body. And as we know, once you start burning fat, good things happen!

Usually, the only negative side effect of intermittent fasting is hunger. Most people experience this side effect only in the first few days while adjusting to the method. But intermittent fasting is not advised for the following people:

- Anyone struggling with or prone to an eating disorder
- Anyone who has issues with blood sugar regulation
- Anyone who suffers from hypoglycemia or diabetes
- Anyone who is malnourished
- Children under 18 years old
- Pregnant women
- Breastfeeding women
- Anyone taking daily medications that must be consumed with food

BENEFITS OF INTERMITTENT FASTING

Healing. Taking long breaks between meals gives your digestive system a break because it isn't actively trying to process and break down food. This break allows your body to rest and heal.

Weight loss. As described above, intermittent fasting can help you lose weight and belly fat.

Simplified meal planning. Most intermittent fasters skip breakfast, meaning that is one less meal to have to plan, prepare, and eat, which saves you time and money.

Intermittent Fasting and Keto in Action

Three of the weekly Clean Keto Lifestyle Meal Plans that follow in the next chapter utilize the 16/8 method of intermittent fasting. This method requires restricting your daily eating period to 8 hours and fasting for 16 hours in between. I find that having an eating window between 11 a.m. and 7 p.m. each day works really well for my clients. But this window can easily be moved, depending on what works best for your own schedule.

During the fasting period, you can still consume water, unsweetened tea, black coffee, and bone broth.

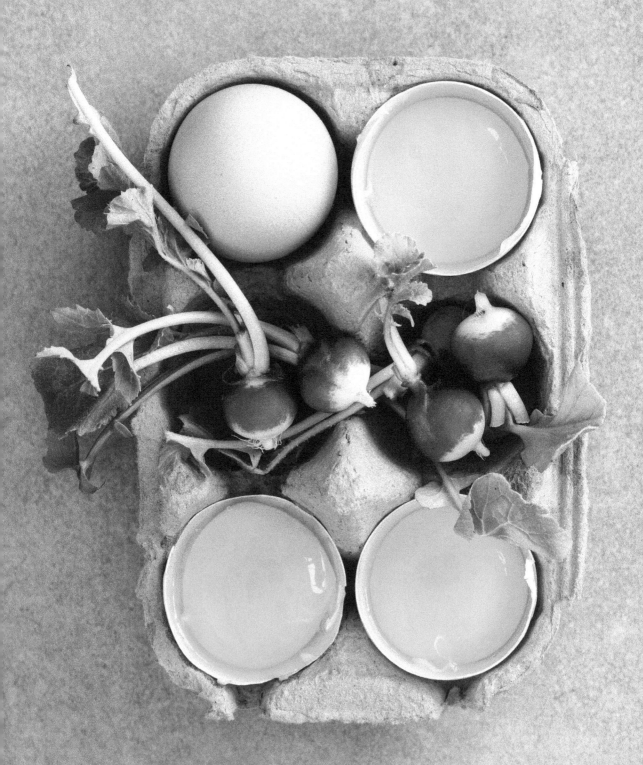

3

CLEAN KETO MEAL PLANS

One of the biggest challenges when starting a ketogenic diet is just that: starting. Many people find themselves stressing out over how to eat 75 percent fat each day, how to avoid carbs, and how to find keto recipes that they'll actually want to eat. I am here to help!

I have done all the work for you, specifically curating five weeks of nourishing (and delicious) keto meal plans, shopping lists, and meal prep instructions intended to minimize your time in the kitchen.

My customized Clean Keto Lifestyle (CKL) meal plans are comprised of only real foods—nothing artificial or processed—and they are designed to turn your body into a lean, mean, fat-burning machine!

These meal plans are great for everyone, no matter your experience with keto or your skill level in the kitchen. They are perfect for those of you who are just starting the keto diet and looking for a fast and straightforward way to incorporate the diet into your life immediately. Or you can simply use the meal plans as a guide to figure out how to structure your meals or get some new recipe inspiration.

A few of my meal plans incorporate intermittent fasting (as discussed in the previous chapter) and thus contain two meals a day, not three.

Keto Tips to Live By

I give all of my clients these tips before they start a keto diet.

DRINK YOUR H₂O

- Drink lots of water! As a minimum, each day, drink at least a half ounce for each pound that you weigh.

- Always start your day with a large glass of water. I like to fill a glass up the night before and set it on my bathroom sink. That way, the next morning when I wake up and head to the bathroom, I have my glass already there, waiting for me.

- If you are following a workout plan and/or sweating, make sure to add even more water to your routine (at least another 24 ounces).

- To keep your electrolytes in balance, sprinkle a small amount of pink Himalayan salt into your water.

AVOID ARTIFICIAL SWEETENERS

- Throw out artificial sweeteners (Splenda, Equal, Sweet'n Low, even Truvia) and anything else that contains aspartame, sucralose, etc. That also means all diet soda.

- These artificial sweeteners are chemicals developed in labs, which are dangerous to your health and also confuse your body. It is hard for your body to tell the difference between artificial sweeteners and actual sugar, so it responds in the same way by raising your blood sugar and insulin levels—hello "glu-coaster!"

- Opt for small amounts (less than 10 grams a day) of pure and unrefined stevia, which comes from a plant and has less impact on your blood sugar levels.

BRACE YOURSELF FOR KETO FLU

- Don't worry—you are not really sick. Keto flu can occur when your body is transitioning its energy source from glucose to fat/ketones. Symptoms can include headaches, nausea, fatigue, irritability, constipation, and soreness. Essentially, you will feel like you have the flu for a few days.

- Be patient. It will go away. Feeling this way is actually a sign that you are getting into ketosis.

- To combat keto flu, or to attempt to avoid it altogether, stay hydrated. Increase the amount of water you are drinking by 16 to 24 ounces and sprinkle pink Himalayan salt into it, drink bone broth, do light exercise, get plenty of sleep, and add additional fats to your meals.

- Most importantly—stay strong! Once you get through this transition phase, you'll be reaping all the amazing benefits of being in ketosis.

SALT YOUR FOOD

Contrary to popular belief, our bodies need salt. Salt helps regulate blood pressure, pass nutrients through our cells, and extract excess acidity in the body.

But not all salts are created equal . . .

Let's first talk about table salt, which is a refined salt that looks like white crystals and is found at most restaurants and probably even in your very own kitchen. This type of salt goes through a commercial process where it is bleached, heated, and infused with chemical anticaking agents. During the process, it is also stripped of its minerals. I say, ditch it!

Upgrade to pink Himalayan salt instead. Pink Himalayan salt is mined from ancient sea beds and is one of the purest salts you can find. Not only is it unrefined, but it also contains a plethora of trace minerals and elements. Pink Himalayan salt is a great source of electrolytes, and when it is combined with water, it provides faster hydration. Hydration and your electrolyte balance is crucial when you are on the ketogenic diet.

Other potential benefits of pink Himalayan salt include:

- Muscle cramp reduction
- Hormone support
- Sleep improvement

Make sure you salt everything to maintain your electrolyte balance. I recommend a teaspoon of pink Himalayan salt a day. All that said, please check with your doctor about salt consumption if you are over 50 or have elevated blood pressure, diabetes, or any other medical condition.

Meal Plan Notes

SERVINGS GUIDANCE

- Most recipes in this book make one serving, but check each individual recipe to be sure.

- On Wednesday nights, you will make a double batch of dinner for leftovers the next day. Simply double all the ingredients in the recipe when cooking. (The shopping lists already account for these double batches.)

- Adjust recipe measurements accordingly if cooking for more people.

FOOD STORAGE

- Some recipes call for half a lemon or lime. Store the remaining half face-down on a small plate in the refrigerator to save for the next use.

- Store fresh herbs in a glass jar filled halfway with water in the refrigerator.

- Some recipes call for 1 cup of coconut milk (most cans have 2½ cups). If a recipe calls for less than 1 can of coconut milk, follow these steps:

  + Shake the can vigorously before opening to blend the solids and the water completely.
  + Open the can and measure out the amount needed.
  + Pour the remaining milk into a sealed container and store it in the refrigerator for up to 5 days.
  + Bonus: Store 1 or 2 cans of coconut milk in the refrigerator at all times so you'll always have a cold can when you want to make a smoothie.

BREAKFAST IS OPTIONAL

- Feel free to omit Meal #1 each day or drink Creamy Coffee (page 158) the whole week as breakfast.

- If you do choose this option, don't forget to remove the breakfast meal ingredients from your weekly shopping list.

MAKING SUBSTITUTIONS

- If you don't like certain foods, just swap them out with an equivalent macronutrient (i.e., chicken for salmon or broccoli for asparagus).

- Make sure to adjust the cooking time and recipe instructions accordingly when making any substitutions.

- If you don't tolerate dairy, you can remove it from the recipes or swap it for a different healthy fat that would work in the recipe.

MORE QUICK TIPS

- Don't binge or stuff yourself. Eat until you are 80 percent full and not to the point of discomfort.

- Coconut oil, avocado oil, ghee, and grass-fed butter are all interchangeable when using for sautéing or roasting. Avoid cooking with extra-virgin olive oil because of its low smoke point.

- If you work during the week, assemble or make your lunch the night before. Keep any dressing on the side—don't pour it over the dish until you are ready to serve.

For each meal plan that follows, make sure to check out the reference table below for what pantry items you will need for the week.

PANTRY STAPLES

FATS	Keto Beginner	Time Saver	Keto & IF	Fat Burner	Maintenance
Avocado oil	√	√	√	√	√
Coconut oil	√		√		√
Extra-virgin olive oil	√	√	√	√	√
Full-fat coconut milk (keep 4 cans on hand)	√	√	√		
Ghee/grass-fed butter	√	√	√	√	√
MCT oil	√	√			
Sesame oil	√		√	√	

CONDIMENTS/SAUCES	Keto Beginner	Time Saver	Keto & IF	Fat Burner	Maintenance
Apple cider vinegar	√	√	√		√
Balsamic vinegar	√			√	√
Beef broth		√			
Coconut aminos	√	√	√	√	√
Chicken broth			√	√	
Diced tomatoes (8-ounce can)			√	√	
Dijon mustard	√		√	√	√
Mayonnaise (no sugar added)		√			
Pure vanilla extract	√	√			
Red wine vinegar	√		√		
Tomato sauce (12-ounce can)		√	√	√	√
Tomato paste		√	√		
Yellow mustard		√			

NUTS/SEEDS	Keto Beginner	Time Saver	Keto & IF	Fat Burner	Maintenance
Almond flour			√		
Chia seeds		√			
Raw chopped pecans		√			√
Raw sliced almonds		√	√	√	
Raw whole almonds					√

DRIED SPICES	Keto Beginner	Time Saver	Keto & IF	Fat Burner	Maintenance
Basil	√		√	√	√
Cayenne pepper		√			
Chili powder	√	√	√		√
Cumin	√	√	√		√
Garlic powder	√	√	√	√	√
Ground black pepper	√	√	√	√	√
Onion powder	√		√		√
Oregano	√	√	√	√	√
Paprika	√	√	√		√
Pink Himalayan salt	√	√	√	√	√
Red pepper flakes	√		√	√	√
Rosemary	√		√	√	√
Thyme	√		√	√	√

POWDER	Keto Beginner	Time Saver	Keto & IF	Fat Burner	Maintenance
Cacao powder	√				
Coffee (ideally organic)	√	√			
Collagen powder	√				
Green tea/matcha tea (ideally organic)	√				
Pure organic stevia (drops/powder)	√	√			

When you are in ketosis, your hunger hormones are regulated, so you don't experience the sudden urges to eat or feel the need to snack between meals. I recommend that my clients try to avoid snacking during the day and only focus on eating balanced meals.

Why is this important? Your body can't burn fat when it is busy digesting food. The more times you eat during the day, the less time your body has to burn fat. That being said, when you're first starting the keto diet, you may need a few snacks to get you through the transition. Here are some of my go-to keto snacks:

- Cucumbers with Keto Ranch (page 91)
- Celery with almond butter
- Avocado drizzled with extra-virgin olive oil and pink Himalayan salt
- Handful of macadamia nuts
- Cup of Bone Broth (page 162)

Keto for Vegetarians and Vegans

Many people think that the ketogenic diet is for meat eaters only, but there are plenty of plant-based fats and proteins that fit perfectly into a Clean Keto Lifestyle. The trick is finding options that are low in carbohydrates. Let's break down the strategy.

FATS

Since fat makes up 75 percent of your daily food intake, fill up your meals with lots of delicious plant-based sources. I have listed my favorite fat sources below. Cook with them, make salad dressings and marinades with them, and top off your meals with them.

- Avocados/avocado oil
- Cocoa butter
- Coconut cream
- Coconut oil
- Flaxseed oil
- Macadamia oil
- MCT oil
- Extra-virgin olive oil
- Olives
- Red palm oil

PROTEINS

Sources of protein for vegetarians and vegans can be a little trickier, because most protein-rich vegan foods also happen to be relatively high in carbohydrates, such as beans, lentils, and grains. Here are some protein sources that are also low in carbs:

- Almonds/almond flour
- Chia seed
- Flaxseed
- Hemp seeds
- Pecans
- Protein powder (pea, hemp, rice—read the labels to ensure that there is no added sugar and that the carb content is low)
- Pumpkin seeds
- Spirulina
- Sunflower seeds
- Tofu (make sure it is organic, unflavored, and non-GMO)
- Walnuts

Adequate protein is vital for your body to function properly, so listen to your body and feed it what it needs. I have worked with some vegan clients who, soon after starting the keto diet, began to crave animal protein. In those cases, I suggested they start with the following options:

Local, pastured eggs. Source them at your farmers' market to get the best nutritional profile, which should include choline, omega-3s, iron, zinc, and protein.

Oysters and mussels. These bivalves are packed with protein, as well as omega-3s. They are also believed to have no central nervous system and are therefore not capable of registering pain.

VEGETABLES

The meal plans and recipes included in this book are full of a wide variety of fresh, colorful vegetables that make the perfect base for vegans and vegetarians alike. Not all of the recipes in the book are free from meat or other animal products, but most of them can be adjusted easily to fit your dietary preference. Here are my go-to strategies for turning any recipe into a plant-based one:

- Swap out grass-fed butter or ghee for coconut oil
- Swap out heavy cream or dairy-based milks for coconut milk or nut milks
- Swap out animal protein for tofu, nuts, or seeds
- Use olives and avocado as toppings in lieu of dairy
- When in doubt, make a keto smoothie using a plant-based protein powder

Meal Plan 1

KETO BEGINNER PLAN

This is my keto beginner meal plan filled with recipes that will keep you satiated all day. It contains a wide variety of flavors and is designed to transition your body into ketosis. Enjoy!

Shopping List

Reminder: The list below has enough ingredients for one person. Increase the quantities accordingly if you are cooking for more people.

PROTEIN
- Bacon (4 slices)
- Boneless chicken thighs (5)
- Eggs (7)
- Ground turkey (6 ounces)
- Pork tenderloin (12 ounces)
- Prosciutto (2 slices)
- Salmon (6-ounce fillet)
- Scallops (6 ounces)
- Shrimp (6 ounces)
- Skirt steak (6 ounces)
- Tuna (5-ounce can packed in olive oil)

VEGETABLES
- Asparagus (14 spears)
- Broccoli (1 medium head)
- Cauliflower (1 head)
- Cherry tomatoes (20)
- Lacinato kale (½ bunch)
- Mixed greens (6 cups)
- Red onion (¾ medium size)
- Scallions (4)
- Spinach (4½ cups)

HERBS
- Cilantro (1 bunch)
- Garlic (14 cloves)
- Ginger root (2-inch piece)

FRUIT
- Avocados (3)
- Blueberries (¼ cup)
- Kalamata olives (4)
- Lemons (2)
- Lime (1)

DAIRY
- Cream cheese (¼ cup)

DAY	MEAL 1	MEAL 2	MEAL 3
MONDAY	Creamy Coffee	Chef Salad	Lemon Salmon & Asparagus
TUESDAY	Chocolate Protein Shake	Shrimp & Avocado Salad	Pork Tenderloin & Cauliflower Mash
WEDNESDAY	Green Tea Latte	Italian Tuna Salad	Balsamic Chicken *Make a double batch*
THURSDAY	Berry Cheesecake Smoothie	Leftover Balsamic Chicken	Pan-Fried Scallops & Garlicky Kale
FRIDAY	Green Smoothie	Spinach Bacon Salad	Beef & Broccoli
SATURDAY	Creamy Coffee	Eggs & Bacon	Turkey Taco Bowl
SUNDAY	Green Tea Latte	Prosciutto Egg Cups	Pork Fried Rice

SUNDAY MEAL PREP

Here is the most efficient way to meal prep on the weekend to minimize your time in the kitchen during the week:

PREPARE THE VEGETABLES

1. Chop the broccoli into florets.
2. Chop the cauliflower into florets.
3. Dice one half of the red onion and chop the remaining quarter into half-inch pieces.
4. Finely slice the scallions.
5. Store all of the above in separate sealed containers in the refrigerator.

COOK AHEAD

1. Preheat the oven to 375°F.
2. Bake the chicken: Season one chicken thigh with salt and freshly ground black pepper, and bake for 30 minutes or until the juices run clear. Let cool, and store in a container in the refrigerator. You will use this thigh for the Chef Salad (page 122).
3. Hard-boil the eggs: While the chicken is baking, place two eggs in a small saucepan and add enough cold water to cover the eggs by several inches. On the stovetop over high heat, bring the water to a gentle boil, and let it boil for 1 minute. Immediately remove the saucepan from the heat, and let the eggs sit in the hot water for an additional 12 minutes. Drain the eggs and rinse them under cold water to stop the cooking process. Store them in a container in the refrigerator. Use in the Chef Salad and Spinach Bacon Salad (page 125).

4. Cook the shrimp: Fill the same pot that you cooked the eggs in with water and bring it to a boil. Add the shrimp and cook for 1 to 3 minutes, until the shrimp turn pink and become opaque. Drain the shrimp in a strainer, and immediately rinse them under cold running water until they are cool to the touch. Store in a container in the refrigerator for use in the Shrimp & Avocado Salad (page 120).

5. Cook the bacon: Put two slices of bacon in a small skillet over medium-high heat; cook until crispy, flipping once. Let cool, chop into 1-inch pieces, and store in a sealed container in the refridgerator for use in the Spinach Bacon Salad.

6. Make the Simple Balsamic Vinaigrette (page 89). Store in a container in the refrigerator for use in the Chef Salad and Shrimp & Avocado Salad.

7. Make a half serving of Italian Vinaigrette (page 90). Store in a container in the refrigerator for use in the Italian Tuna Salad.

OPTIONAL: Make the Chef Salad if you will be taking it to work on Monday. Keep the dressing on the side until you are ready to serve.

Meal Plan 2

This meal plan uses major weekend meal prep and lots of leftovers to minimize your time in the kitchen during the week! This is a great plan to use when you know you have a busy week ahead.

Shopping List

Reminder: The list below has enough ingredients for one person. Increase the quantities accordingly if you are cooking for more people.

PROTEIN
- Bacon (14 slices)
- Boneless chicken thighs (4)
- Eggs (6)
- Ground beef (24 ounces)
- Pork tenderloin (6 ounces)
- Salmon (6-ounce fillet)
- Shrimp (12 ounces)
- Skirt steak (6 ounces)

VEGETABLES
- Asparagus (6 spears)
- Broccoli (2 medium heads)
- Cauliflower (1 head)
- Cherry tomatoes (4 count)
- Green bell pepper (¼)
- Green beans (1 pound)
- Mixed greens (2 cups)
- Radishes (2)
- Red bell pepper (½)
- Red onion (¾ medium-size)
- White onion (¾ medium-size)
- Zucchini (1)

HERBS
- Garlic (18 cloves)

FRUIT
- Lemons (3)

DAIRY
- Cheddar cheese (¼ cup cubed)
- Parmesan cheese (1 teaspoon freshly grated)

DAY	MEAL 1	MEAL 2	MEAL 3
MONDAY	Overnight Chia Pudding	Grandma's Broccoli Salad	Slow Cooker Keto Chili
TUESDAY	Creamy Coffee	Leftover Slow Cooker Keto Chili	Bacon-Wrapped Chicken & Cauliflower Mash *Make a double batch*
WEDNESDAY	Overnight Chia Pudding	Leftover Bacon-Wrapped Chicken & Cauliflower Mash	Roasted Shrimp & Veggies *Make a double batch*
THURSDAY	Creamy Coffee	Leftover Roasted Shrimp & Veggies	Cheeseburger Meat Loaf & Southern Green Beans *Make a double batch*
FRIDAY	Overnight Chia Pudding	Leftover Cheeseburger Meat Loaf & Southern Green Beans	Lemon Salmon & Asparagus
SATURDAY	Creamy Coffee	Eggs & Bacon	Pork Tenderloin & Roasted Broccoli
SUNDAY	Green Tea Latte	Eggs & Bacon	Steak Salad

SUNDAY MEAL PREP

Here is the most efficient way to meal prep on the weekend to minimize your time in the kitchen during the week:

PREPARE THE VEGETABLES

1. Chop the broccoli into florets.
2. Chop the cauliflower into florets.
3. Chop the red bell pepper into half-inch pieces.
4. Dice the green bell pepper.
5. Dice a quarter of the red onion and chop the remaining half into half-inch pieces.
6. Dice the white onion.
7. Slice the zucchini into half-moons.
8. Slice the radishes.
9. Trim the ends of the green beans.
10. Store all of the above in separate sealed containers in the refrigerator.

COOK AHEAD

1. Prepare the Slow Cooker Keto Chili (page 129). Simmer for about 3 hours, let cool, and store in a covered container in the refrigerator.
2. Preheat the oven to 400°F.
3. Prepare a double batch of the Bacon-Wrapped Chicken (page 142), and bake it for 25 minutes.
4. Mix up the Cheeseburger Meat Loaf (page 153) while the chicken is baking.
5. Once the Bacon-Wrapped Chicken is finished cooking, take it out of the oven to cool. Place it in a sealed container and put it in the refrigerator.
6. Bake the Cheeseburger Meat Loaf: Place the meat mixture on a baking sheet and shape it into a loaf. Lower the oven temperature to 350°F. Bake for 1 hour or until cooked through.
7. Make Grandma's Broccoli Salad (page 126). Store it overnight in a covered container in the refrigerator to let the flavors develop.
8. Make double batches of the Cauliflower Mash (page 109) and the Southern Green Beans (page 117). Store in separate sealed containers in the refrigerator.
9. Make three servings of the Overnight Chia Pudding (page 101), and store each serving in an individual sealed container in the refrigerator.

Meal Plan 3

KETO AND INTERMITTENT FASTING MEAL PLAN

If you have followed the first two meal plans in this chapter, then congratulations! You should officially be in ketosis. Now let's incorporate some intermittent fasting to complement your keto meals. With this meal plan, I want you to incorporate the 16/8 method of intermittent fasting (see page 28), so that means you will have an eating window of 8 hours (for instance, 11 a.m. to 7 p.m.). Aim to have Meal #1 at 11 a.m. or later each day, and make sure to finish Meal #2 by 7 p.m. The rest of the time outside these feeding hours, you will not be eating, but you can still consume water, black coffee, unsweetened tea, and bone broth. Since you are only having two meals, you should consume an extra 2 servings of fat each day during your eating window in addition to these recipes. You can easily fit them in by using another serving of fat while cooking or you can top your meal with some butter/oil before eating.

Shopping List

Reminder: The following list has enough ingredients for one person. Increase the quantities accordingly if you are cooking for more people.

PROTEIN

- Bacon (4 slices)
- Boneless chicken thighs (6)
- Eggs (8)
- Ground turkey (6 ounces)
- Ground chicken (6 ounces)
- Pork tenderloin (12 ounces)
- Prosciutto (2 slices)
- Rib eye steak (6 ounces)
- Salmon (6-ounce fillet)
- Scallops (6 ounces)

VEGETABLES

- Bibb lettuce leaves (6)
- Broccoli (1 medium head)
- Brussels sprouts (⅓ pound)
- Cauliflower (1½ heads)
- Cherry tomatoes (4)
- Cucumber (¾)
- Green bell pepper (¼)
- Lacinato kale (½ bunch)
- Mixed greens (2 cups)
- Cremini mushrooms (8-ounce package, presliced)
- Red onion (½ medium-size)
- Red bell pepper (¼)
- Scallions (4)
- Spinach (8½ cups)
- White onion (½ medium-size)

HERBS

- Cilantro (1 bunch)
- Garlic (18 cloves)
- Ginger root (3-inch piece)
- Parsley (1 bunch)

FRUIT

- Avocados (2)
- Kalamata olives (4)
- Lemons (1½)
- Lime (1)

DAIRY

- Cream cheese (1 tablespoon)
- Feta cheese (1 tablespoon)
- Grass-fed butter (½ stick)
- Parmesan cheese (3 teaspoons freshly grated)

DAY	MEAL 1	MEAL 2
MONDAY	Chicken Tortilla Soup	Asian-Style Salmon & Roasted Broccoli
TUESDAY	Chopped Salad	Pan-Fried Scallops & Crispy Brussels Sprouts
WEDNESDAY	Leftover Chicken Tortilla Soup	Pork Fried Rice *Make a double batch*
THURSDAY	Leftover Pork Fried Rice	Lettuce-Wrapped Chicken Burger & Asian Spiced Cucumbers
FRIDAY	Spinach Bacon Salad	Turkey Taco Bowl & Mexican Cauliflower Rice
SATURDAY	Prosciutto Egg Cups	Rib-Eye Steak & Roasted Mushrooms & Creamed Spinach
SUNDAY	Eggs & Bacon	Chicken Strip Wraps & Garlicky Kale

SUNDAY MEAL PREP

Here is the most efficient way to meal prep on the weekend to minimize your time in the kitchen during the week:

PREPARE THE VEGETABLES

1. Chop the broccoli into florets.
2. Chop the cauliflower into florets.
3. Chop the cucumber into half-inch pieces.
4. Chop the green bell pepper into half-inch pieces.
5. Chop the red onion into half-inch pieces.
6. Dice the red bell pepper.
7. Dice the white onion.
8. Finely slice the scallions.
9. Finely slice the Brussels sprouts.
10. Store all of the above in separate sealed containers in the refrigerator.

COOK AHEAD

1. Make the Chicken Tortilla Soup (page 128), let it cool, and store it in a sealed container in the refrigerator.
2. Preheat the oven to 375°F.
3. Cook the chicken: Season one chicken thigh with salt and freshly ground black pepper, and bake for 30 minutes or until the juices run clear. Let cool, and store it in a container in the refrigerator. You will use this thigh for the Chopped Salad (page 123).
4. Hard-boil an egg: While the chicken is baking, place one egg in a small saucepan and add enough cold water to cover the egg by several inches. On the stovetop over high heat, bring the water to a gentle boil, and let it boil for 1 minute. Immediately remove the saucepan from the heat and let the egg sit in the hot water for an additional 12 minutes. Drain the egg, and rinse it under cold water to stop the cooking process. Store in a sealed container in the refrigerator. Use in the Spinach Bacon Salad (page 125).
5. Cook the bacon: Put two slices of bacon in a small skillet over medium-high heat, and cook until crispy, flipping once. Let cool, chop into 1-inch pieces, and store in a sealed container in the refrigerator for use in the Spinach Bacon Salad.
6. Make the Garlic & Herb Compound Butter (page 85). Store it in the refrigerator for use in the Rib Eye Steak (page 152) and Roasted Mushrooms (page 112).
7. Make a half serving of the Italian Vinaigrette (page 90). Store in a sealed container in the refrigerator for use in the Chopped Salad.

Meal Plan 4

This Fat Burner Meal Plan also uses the 16/8 method of intermittent fasting (see page 28). As discussed earlier in the book, this powerful combination of the keto diet coupled with a 16-hour fasting window, where you essentially skip breakfast and only eat during an 8-hour window, maximizes your body's ability to burn fat. As a friendly reminder, you need to implement intermittent fasting consistently to reap the benefits of it and continue to see lasting results. Make sure to add in your additional 2 servings of fat each day.

Shopping List

Reminder: The following list has enough ingredients for one person. Increase the quantities accordingly if you are cooking for more people.

PROTEIN

- Bacon (10 slices)
- Boneless chicken thighs (7)
- Chicken tenderloins (3)
- Eggs (5)
- Ground beef (12 ounces)
- Ground pork (6 ounces)
- Ground turkey (6 ounces)
- Salmon (6-ounce fillet)
- Skirt steak (6 ounces)
- Tuna (5-ounce can packed in olive oil)

VEGETABLES

- Asparagus (7 spears)
- Broccoli (1 medium head)
- Brussels sprouts (⅓ pound)
- Cabbage, shredded or cabbage coleslaw mix (2 cups)
- Cauliflower (1 head)
- Cherry tomatoes (16 count)
- Cucumber (¼)
- Green bell pepper (¼)
- Lacinato kale (½ bunch)
- Mixed greens (2 cups)
- Radishes (2)
- Red onion (½ medium-size)
- Scallion (1)
- Spinach (3 cups)
- White onion (¼ medium-size)
- Zucchini (1½)

HERBS

- Garlic (23 cloves)
- Ginger root (2-inch piece)

FRUIT

- Avocado (1½)
- Kalamata olives (8)
- Lemons (1½)
- Lime (1)

DAIRY

- Cheddar cheese
  (1-ounce slice)
- Feta cheese
  (1 tablespoon)
- Goat cheese
  (1 tablespoon)
- Parmesan cheese
  (1 teaspoon
  freshly grated)

DAY	MEAL 1	MEAL 2
MONDAY	Steak Salad	Egg Roll in a Bowl
TUESDAY	Zesty Chicken Tender Salad	Mini Burger Sliders & Crispy Brussels Sprouts
WEDNESDAY	Italian Tuna Salad	Bacon-Wrapped Chicken & Cauliflower Mash *Make a double batch*
THURSDAY	Leftover Bacon-Wrapped Chicken & Cauliflower Mash	Asian-Style Salmon & Galicky Kale
FRIDAY	Chopped Salad	Italian Zoodles
SATURDAY	Eggs with Goat Cheese & Asparagus	Balsamic Chicken
SUNDAY	Eggs & Bacon	Turkey Meatballs & Roasted Broccoli

Here is the most efficient way to meal prep on the weekend to minimize your time in the kitchen during the week:

PREPARE THE VEGETABLES

1. Chop the broccoli into florets.
2. Chop the cauliflower into florets.
3. Chop the cucumber into half-inch pieces.
4. Chop the green bell pepper into half-inch pieces.
5. Chop the red onion into half-inch pieces.
6. Dice the white onion.
7. Finely slice the Brussels sprouts.
8. Finely slice the scallion.
9. Shred the cabbage.
10. Slice the radishes.
11. Store all of the above in separate sealed containers in the refrigerator.

COOK AHEAD

1. Preheat the oven to 375°F.
2. Cook the chicken: Season one chicken thigh and three chicken tenderloins with salt and freshly ground black pepper, and bake for 30 minutes or until the juices run clear. Let cool, and store in a container in the refrigerator. You will use the thigh for the Chopped Salad (page 123) and the tenderloins for the Chicken Tender Salad (page 124).
3. Make a full serving of Italian Vinaigrette (page 90). Store it in the refrigerator in a sealed container for use in the Italian Tuna Salad (page 121) and Chopped Salad (page 123).
4. Make the dressing for the Zesty Chicken Tender Salad and store it in the refrigerator in a sealed container.
5. Make the Steak Salad (page 127) if you will be taking it to work on Monday. Keep the dressing on the side until you are ready to serve.

Meal Plan 5

You did it! By now, you are off the "glu-coaster" and are riding on the ketone highway, so this is the last week of curated CKL meal plans. This meal plan once again incorporates the 16/8 method of intermittent fasting, so don't forget to add in an extra 2 servings of fat to your day. Going forward, feel free to repeat any of the weekly meal plans in the book. I also encourage you to build your own meal plans using the 8-3-6 formula that I discussed earlier (see page 16). As your body gets used to being in ketosis, your macro needs may change. Listen to your body, pay attention to what you are eating and how your body reacts, then adjust accordingly.

Shopping List

Reminder: The following list has enough ingredients for one person. Increase the quantities accordingly if you are cooking for more people.

PROTEIN
- Boneless chicken thighs (5)
- Eggs (6)
- Ground chicken (6 ounces)
- Ground turkey (10 ounces)
- Pork tenderloin (6 ounces)
- Prosciutto (1 slice)
- Salmon (6-ounce fillet)
- Shrimp (6 ounces)
- Skirt steak (18 ounces)
- Tuna (5-ounce can packed in olive oil)

VEGETABLES
- Asparagus (6 spears)
- Bibb lettuce leaves (6)
- Broccoli (2 medium heads)
- Cherry tomatoes (16 count)
- Green beans (½ pound)
- Green bell pepper (¼)
- Mixed greens (4 cups)
- Red onion (1½ medium-size)
- Red bell pepper (½)
- Scallion (1)
- Spinach (½ cup)
- White onion (½ medium-size)
- Yellow summer squash (½)
- Zucchini (1½)

HERBS
- Basil, fresh (3 cups)
- Cilantro (1 bunch)
- Garlic (18 cloves)
- Ginger root (2-inch piece)

FRUIT
- Avocados (3½)
- Kalamata olives (4)
- Lemons (2½)
- Limes (1¼)

DAIRY
- Parmesan cheese (1 teaspoon freshly grated)

DAY	MEAL 1	MEAL 2
MONDAY	Lettuce-Wrapped Chicken Burger	Lemon Salmon & Asparagus
TUESDAY	Italian Tuna Salad	Turkey Taco Bowl
WEDNESDAY	Chicken Strip Wraps & Sautéed Summer Squash	Beef and Broccoli *Make a double batch*
THURSDAY	Leftover Beef & Broccoli	Basil Chicken Zucchini "Pasta"
FRIDAY	Chef Salad	Roasted Shrimp & Veggies
SATURDAY	Turkey Egg Scramble	Pork Tenderloin & Southern Green Beans
SUNDAY	Italian Omelet	Steak Fajitas

SUNDAY MEAL PREP

Here is the most efficient way to meal prep on the weekend to minimize your time in the kitchen during the week:

PREPARE THE VEGETABLES

1. Chop the broccoli into florets.
2. Dice one red onion and chop the additional half into half-inch pieces.
3. Dice one quarter of the red bell pepper and chop the other quarter into half-inch pieces.

4. Dice one quarter of the white onion and slice the other quarter into thin, fajita-style strips.
5. Finely slice the scallion.
6. Slice the green bell pepper into thin, fajita-style strips.
7. Slice one whole zucchini into half-moons (save the other half to be spiralized later in the week).
8. Slice the yellow summer squash into half-moons.
9. Trim the ends of the green beans.
10. Store all of the above in separate sealed containers in the refrigerator.

COOK AHEAD
1. Preheat the oven to 375°F.
2. Cook the chicken: Season one chicken thigh with salt and freshly ground black pepper, and bake for 30 minutes or until the juices run clear. Let cool, and store in the refrigerator. You will use it for the Chef Salad Chef Salad (page 122) during the week.
3. Hard-boil an egg: While the chicken is baking, place one egg in a small saucepan and add enough cold water to cover the egg by several inches. On the stovetop over high heat, bring the water to a gentle boil, and let it boil for 1 minute. Immediately remove the saucepan from the heat, and let the egg sit in the hot water for an additional 12 minutes. Drain the egg and rinse it under cold water to stop the cooking process. Store it in a sealed container in the refrigerator. Use in the Chef Salad.
4. Make a half serving of the Italian Vinaigrette (page 90). Store it in the refrigerator in a sealed container for the Italian Tuna Salad (page 121).
5. Make a half serving of the Simple Balsamic Vinaigrette (page 89). Store it in the refrigerator in a sealed container for the Chef Salad.
6. Make the Basil Pesto (page 87). Store it in the refrigerator in a sealed container for the Basil Chicken Zucchini "Pasta" (page 139) and Italian Omelet (page 100).
7. Make the Lettuce-Wrapped Chicken Burger (page 136) if you will be taking it to work on Monday. Don't assemble the burger or slice the avocado until you are ready to serve.

As you go through your own personal keto journey and these 5 weeks of meal plans, you will inevitably have questions. Here are the most popular questions I get from my clients.

How do I know if I am in ketosis? The most popular ways to test are blood, breath, or urine.

- **Blood Ketone Testing:** In my opinion, testing the blood for beta-hydroxybutyrate (i.e., ketones) is the most accurate approach. You can buy a Blood Ketone Meter for around $25 to 60 with individual strips costing about $4 each. Test your levels in the morning and night (ideally the same time each day). You are aiming for a range of 0.5 to 3.0 mmol/L, which means you are in nutritional ketosis. Don't get discouraged if it takes a few weeks to hit this range. Everyone's body is different. The important thing is to not give up and continue fueling your body the CKL way!
- **Breath Ketone Testing:** Another method for testing your ketone levels is through your breath. You can purchase a Breath Ketone Meter that will test for the presence of the Acetone, which is a ketone body. While not quite as reliable, this type of meter is cheaper than a Blood Ketone Meter and doesn't involve pricking your finger!
- **Urine Strip Testing:** Urine strips are not as accurate because they only test for excess ketone bodies that are excreted through the urine, rather than giving you insight to what is going on in your blood. However, they do give you some indication of your ketone levels when you first start the keto diet and are an inexpensive option.

What supplements should I take? What one body needs can vary drastically from what another needs, so in general supplements should be personalized and tailored for each individual. That said, there are a few standard supplements that I recommend to my clients and that I personally use.

- **Pink Himalayan salt:** Add it to your beverages, cook with it, and season your food with it to balance and restore your electrolytes.
- **Magnesium:** Magnesium deficiency can be common on keto, so supplementing is a good idea. Look for a good quality brand that has no added sugar.
- **Probiotics:** Probiotics are a requirement! You need this friendly gut-bacteria to ensure your digestive system is happy and healthy. I drink a tablespoon of sauerkraut juice or apple cider vinegar each day. I also take a probiotic capsule daily.
- **MCT or Fish Oil:** Keto is all about the fats, so adding a regular dose of them in a convenient supplement form is a great daily habit. Look for organic MCT oil and the cleanest brand of fish oil.

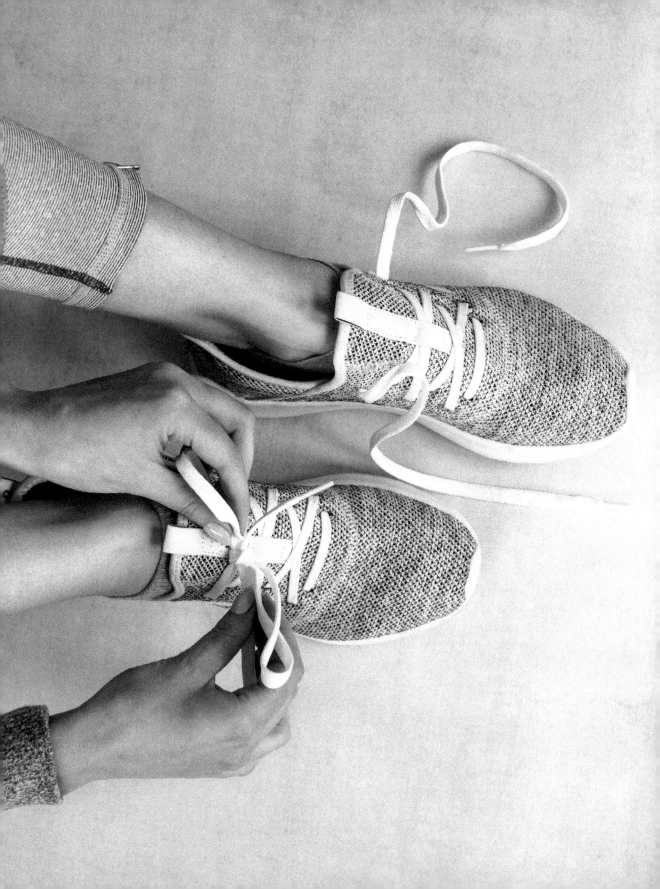

Chapter

4

EXERCISE

P roper nutrition and diet are definitely the biggest factors when it comes
to your heath, but moving your body also plays an important role. Exercise
can be a controversial topic. Some people love it, others detest it. Some
exercise too much, while others don't do it enough. This chapter is focused on
breaking down the facts and giving you an effective workout plan that will perfectly complement a ketogenic diet.

Exercise on Keto

"Is it possible to work out without eating carbs?" is a popular question I get from my clients. The answer is an unequivocal yes! It all goes back to science and how the body works, so let's break it down.

- As you know by now, the body will use glucose as its main fuel source by default.

- A portion of the glucose that isn't burned immediately is converted to glycogen and stored primarily in the liver and muscles for future use (the rest is converted to triglycerides and stored in your fat cells). When you are working out, this stored glycogen provides fuel for the body as needed.

- When your body enters ketosis, it is able to access stored fat for energy and rely less on glycogen as a fuel source when exercising.

- Because of your ability to use your own body fat efficiently for fuel while on the ketogenic diet, you won't need to tap into glycogen stores that often.

What does all this mean? It means that your body doesn't need carbs to be able to exercise effectively. Instead, it will find a way to use what it already has as an energy source to ensure that you have successful workouts.

Build a Plan that Works for You

For decades, people have been told to eat less and exercise more in order to lose weight, which is proving to be very bad advice. In fact, overexercising or consistently pushing your body too hard, too long, or too often can do more harm than good by putting too much stress on your body. This stress can stall weight loss, create carb cravings, and drive excess insulin production.

On the other hand, failing to adequately move your body and spending too much time in a sedentary state can lead to health issues and weight gain, as well. Your body needs to move, and when you don't move it, your risk for disease increases.

What is the right answer? Just like the ketogenic diet takes cues from our ancestors when it comes to what and how often we eat, the same goes for exercise. That means living an active lifestyle full of consistent movement focused on a combination of low-impact cardio and shorter, high-intensity workouts.

Regular physical movement is a fantastic way to support metabolic function, improve digestion, lift your mood, and boost your energy. The great news is that you don't need to spend hours a day in the gym to see results. Let's break down the CKL Exercise Strategy.

- **Low-Impact Cardio:** Every day, focus on consistent movement and make it a priority to fit in as much as possible.
  + Go for refreshing walks in the mornings and evenings with your family, your friends, or your dog.
  + Park in the farthest spot from the entrance.
  + Take the stairs instead of the elevator.
  + Pace around while talking on the phone.
  + Go to a yoga or Pilates class.
  + Play with your kids.
  + Stretch and do yoga poses while watching TV.

- **Shorter, High-Intensity Workout:** 3 or 4 days a week, focus on 30 minutes of high-intensity workouts.
  + Sprint intervals
  + HIIT workouts
  + Dance cardio
  + Swimming
  + Cycling

That's it! A simple and straightforward approach to fitness. The secret to success is to make sure you're doing the type of exercise that you and your body love. If you hate your workout, it's going to be a lot more difficult to maintain consistency.

Pick a routine that works for your personality type. Variation is great for some people, while others enjoy doing the same type of exercise every day. Try different approaches to see what works best for you and what you can really stick to.

What to Know Before Your Workout

1. Stretch before and after you exercise.
2. Drink plenty of water, especially if you are sweating. Add a pinch of pink Himalayan salt to balance your electrolytes.
3. If you're in serious pain, don't force yourself to work out.
4. Take Epsom salt baths after you work out. Epsom salts are anti-inflammatory and detoxifying.
5. Change your perspective. Look at exercise as a celebration of your body's ability to move, not something that you feel forced to do or dread doing.

Workout Plan

I developed this "Toned and Tight Plan" to work in conjunction with the keto diet so you can maximize your results. The workout program uses high-intensity interval training (HIIT), which is a form of exercise where you perform quick bursts of exercise at 100 percent effort and intensity and then follow these bursts with short recovery periods. By training in this manner, you keep your heart rate up and are able to burn more fat in less time.

THE BENEFITS OF HIIT

Increases your metabolism. The powerful combination of high-intensity effort coupled with interval-style training speeds up your metabolic rate, which gives your body a metabolism boost well after you have completed your workout. In fact, this boost can last up to 48 hours, meaning that you are burning fat well after you've finished your workout!

Quick and convenient. HIIT workouts are usually 30 minutes or less and can be done anywhere, including the privacy of your own home, in a hotel room when you are traveling, outside in a park, or at your local gym.

No need for fancy equipment. You don't have dumbbells or belong to a gym? No problem! High-intensity interval workouts mostly consist of exercises that use your body weight rather than any special equipment, which makes them very convenient and mobile.

Do as many reps as you can for one minute of each of the exercises below (resting for 15 to 30 seconds between each exercise). Repeat the entire circuit 4 times.

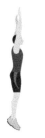

ONE MINUTE JUMPING JACKS
- Start in a standing position with your feet together and your arms by your sides.
- Jump your feet out to the side while simultaneously raising your hands over your head.
- Immediately jump back to the starting position.
- Repeat this sequence in a rhythmic motion.

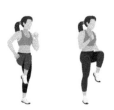

ONE MINUTE HIGH KNEES
- Start in a standing position with your feet hip-distance apart and your arms by your sides.
- Lift one knee toward your chest as high as possible while raising your opposite arm in a runner's position.
- Return to the starting position and quickly lift the other knee and arm in the same manner.
- Repeat this sequence in a fast motion.
- Advanced Option: Jump as you lift each knee to your chest.

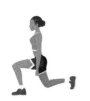

ONE MINUTE BACK LUNGES (30 SECONDS EACH LEG)
- Start in a standing position with your feet hip-distance apart and your hands on your hips.
- With your right foot, take a large step backward, bending your knee at a 90-degree angle so your shin is parallel to the ground.
- Push off your right foot to return to the starting position.
- Repeat the movement with the same leg for 30 seconds; switch to the other leg and perform the exercise for an additional 30 seconds.

ONE MINUTE TRICEP DIPS

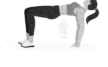

- Sit on the floor with your knees bent in front of you and your feet flat on the ground.
- Position your arms behind your back, with your palms on the floor and your fingers pointing toward your body.
- Slowly lift your hips toward the ceiling so your butt is no longer touching the ground and you are in a tabletop position.
- While maintaining this position, gently bend your elbows and then straighten them.
- Repeat this bend and straighten movement for 20 seconds. Rest briefly, and repeat 2 more times.

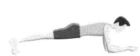

ONE MINUTE FOREARM PLANK HOLD

- Lie facedown on the ground.
- Lift yourself up to balance on your forearms (your forearms should be touching the ground) and your toes.
- Make sure your elbows are directly under your shoulders, your back is straight, your navel is pulled in, and your head is looking down at the ground. Imagine creating a straight line from your shoulders to your feet.
- Hold this position as long as you can, gently lower yourself to the ground, and then repeat.
- Advanced Option: Rather than balancing on your forearms, straighten your arms while keeping your hands directly underneath your shoulders to resemble a push-up position. Make sure to keep your back straight and your core tight.

DAY 2

If the weather permits, head outside! Go for a long walk or leisurely bike ride for at least 45 minutes. Here are some benefits of exercising outside:

- Outdoor exercise lifts your mood.
- You breathe cleaner air outside.
- It's good for your mental health to disconnect and be in nature.

Do as many reps as you can for one minute of each of the exercises below (resting for 15 to 30 seconds between each exercise). Repeat the entire circuit 4 times.

ONE MINUTE BUTT KICKS (ALTERNATING LEGS)

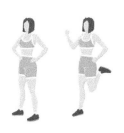

- Start in a standing position with your feet hip-distance apart and your hands on your hips.
- Lift one of your heels towards your butt while raising your opposite arm in a runner's position.
- Aim to make contact with your butt, and then return your heel to the ground and repeat on the other leg.
- Repeat this alternating sequence as quickly as you can.

ONE MINUTE SIDE SQUAT KICKS (ALTERNATING LEGS)

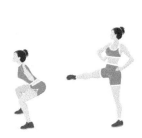

- Start in a standing position with your feet hip-distance apart and your hands on your hips.
- Keeping your weight in your heels, bend your knees and lower your hips into a squat position.
- Rise back up to a standing position and, while squeezing your butt, lift one of your legs to the side, keeping it straight with your knee facing forward.
- Return to a standing position and repeat, lifting your other leg to the side.
- Repeat this sequence, and continue alternating legs.

ONE MINUTE LUNGES (ALTERNATING LEGS)

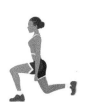

- Start in a standing position with your feet hip-distance apart and your hands on your hips.
- Keeping your torso upright, take a large step forward with your right foot.
- Slowly bend your right knee into a 90-degree angle, making sure to keep your knee directly over your ankle.
- Hold this position for 3 seconds, and then push off your right foot and return to the starting position.
- Repeat the same lunge movement with your left leg.
- Repeat this sequence, and continue alternating legs.

ONE MINUTE Ys & Ts (ALTERNATING 10 SECONDS FOR EACH EXERCISE)

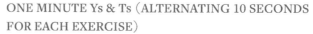
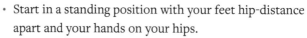

- Start in a standing position with your feet hip-distance apart and your hands on your hips.
- Lift and straighten your arms overhead into a Y position and hold for 10 seconds.
- Keeping your arms straight, lower your arms to shoulder height so they are in a T position; hold for 10 seconds.
- After 10 seconds, raise your arms back up into a Y position.
- Continue alternating your arms between the Y and T positions with no breaks for 1 minute.

ONE MINUTE PLANK TO HAND WALK UPS

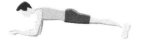
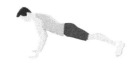

- Lie facedown on the ground.
- Lift yourself up to balance on your forearms (your forearms should be touching the ground) and your toes.
- Make sure your elbows are directly under your shoulders, your back is straight, your navel is pulled in, and your head is looking down at the ground. Imagine creating a straight line from your shoulders to your feet.
- Without changing your body position, lift up from your right elbow to straighten your right arm and place your right hand on the ground.
- Do the same movement with your left arm, so you end up in a push-up position; hold this position for 3 seconds.
- Bending one arm at a time, return to balancing on your forearms.
- Continue to repeat this "walk up" sequence.

DAY 4

Go for a long walk or leisurely bike ride for at least 45 minutes.

Do as many reps as you can for one minute of each exercise below (resting for 15 to 30 seconds between each exercise). Repeat the entire circuit 4 times.

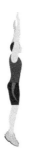

ONE MINUTE JUMPING JACKS

- Start in a standing position with your feet together and your arms by your sides.
- Jump your feet out to the side while simultaneously raising your hands over your head.
- Immediately jump back to the starting position.
- Repeat this sequence in a rhythmic motion.

ONE MINUTE SINGLE LEG GLUTE BRIDGE (ALTERNATING LEGS)

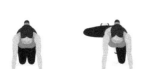

- Start on all fours with your knees bent underneath your hips and your arms directly under your shoulders, elbows slightly bent, and your palms flat on the floor.
- Lift one leg to the side until it is parallel to the ground, keeping your knee bent at a 90-degree angle.
- Squeeze your butt and lower your knee to the starting position.
- Repeat the same movement using your other leg.
- Continue to alternate lifting each leg.

ONE MINUTE BIRD DOG (30 SECONDS EACH LEG)

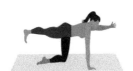

- Start on all fours with your knees bent underneath your hips and your arms directly under your shoulders, elbows slightly bent, and your palms flat on the floor.
- Keeping your core tight, reach your left arm forward, keeping it straight and parallel to the ground, and simultaneously press and straighten your right leg back with your heel flexed. Make sure to keep your hips parallel to the ground the entire time.
- Tightening your abs, return to the starting position; repeat the movement on the same leg for 30 seconds.
- After 30 seconds, repeat the same exercise on the opposite side.

ONE MINUTE SHOULDER TAPS

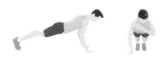

- Lie facedown on the ground.
- Lift yourself up, straightening your arms and keeping your hands directly underneath your shoulders in a push-up position.
- Make sure to keep your back straight and your core tight.
- Lift your left hand off the ground, bend your arm, and tap your right shoulder.
- Return your hand to the floor and repeat the same movement with your right hand.
- Keep alternating hands while remaining in this position.

ONE MINUTE BOAT POSE

- Sit on the ground with your knees bent and feet flat on the floor.
- Grab the back of your thighs with your hands and, keeping your abs tight, slowly start to lean back to allow your feet to come off the ground.
- While leaning back slightly, lift your feet toward the ceiling until your shins are parallel to the floor.
- Hold this position and, with your palms facing up, extend your arms in front of you at shoulder height.
- Straighten your legs upward so your body creates a V shape.
- Hold this position for 10 seconds.
- Slowly return to the starting position and repeat.

DAY 6

Go for a long walk or leisurely bike ride for at least 45 minutes.

Do as many reps as you can for one minute of each of the exercises below (resting for 15 to 30 seconds between each exercise). Repeat the entire circuit 4 times.

ONE MINUTE SQUAT JUMPS

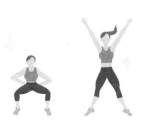

- Start in a standing position with your feet hip-distance apart and your hands on your hips.
- Keeping your weight in your heels, bend your knees and lower your hips into a squat position.
- Jump up toward the ceiling and land back in a squat position.
- Repeat jumping and squatting in a continuous motion.

ONE MINUTE PULSE LUNGES (30 SECONDS EACH LEG)

- Start in a standing position with your feet hip-distance apart and your hands on your hips.
- Keeping your torso upright, take a large step forward with your right foot.
- Slowly bend your right knee into a 90-degree angle, making sure to keep your knee directly over your ankle.
- In this lunge position, begin pulsing up and down, lifting your torso up 2 to 3 inches and then back down. Pulse for 30 seconds.
- Return to the starting position and repeat the same lunge and pulsing movement with your other leg for an additional 30 seconds.

ONE MINUTE MOUNTAIN CLIMBERS

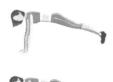

- Lie facedown on the ground.
- Lift yourself up, straightening your arms and keeping your hands directly underneath your shoulders in a push-up position.
- Bring your right knee up to your chest, not allowing your toes to touch the ground, and quickly return your foot back to the starting position.

- Next, immediately bring your left knee up to your chest and return it back to the starting position, like you are running in place.
- Keep doing this running-like motion for 60 seconds.

ONE MINUTE SUPERMANS

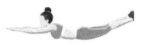

- Lie facedown on the ground with your arms stretched out over your head and your legs straight, resting the tops of your feet on the floor, toes pointed.
- Simultaneously, lift your arms, head, chest, and legs off the floor a few inches; hold for 3 seconds. Your body position should resemble Superman flying.
- Gently return to the starting position, and repeat.

ONE MINUTE FLUTTER KICKS

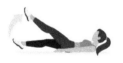
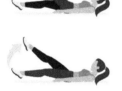

- Lie down on your back with your legs straight, arms at your sides with your palms on the ground.
- Keeping your lower back on the ground, tighten your abs and lift your feet 6 inches off the floor, keeping your legs straight.
- Begin alternating your legs up and down in a flutter-like motion for 15 seconds.
- Lower both legs to the ground, rest, and repeat the exercise 3 more times.

TREAT YOURSELF

We all do it. At some point we push ourselves too hard. Whether it's at the gym or at work, it's easy to lose sight of the most important thing—taking care of ourselves. If you don't prioritize your health and well-being first, you are doing a disservice to not only your body and your mind—but also to your spouse, your kids, your friends, your co-workers, and anyone else who depends on you.

The key is to recognize when you are neglecting your self-care and then take actions to give yourself the love you need and deserve. Setting aside time for yourself is critical for your physical and emotional wellness, and it is a nonnegotiable when it comes to a Clean Keto Lifestyle.

Here are my favorite self-care methods:

- Take a relaxing bath
- Journal for 15 minutes
- Do a guided meditation
- Take a walk outside with the sole intention of soaking up nature's beauty
- Pamper yourself at the spa or get a massage

The goal is to give your body a much needed break to allow it to rest and replenish. Don't look at these self-care activities as frivolous or selfish; instead look at them as essential for your health.

Experiment with different self-care techniques, and see what works best for you. The more you give to yourself in terms of self-care, the more you will be able to give to others.

5

KEEPING KETO WHILE YOU ARE OUT & ABOUT

This book is called *Clean Keto Lifestyle* for a reason—my goal is to make eating quality foods based on ketogenic diet principles a lasting and amazing way of life for anyone. One of the biggest challenges individuals face when it comes to making this a reality is successfully navigating social situations.

Our culture is largely centered around food—think happy hours, holidays, family gatherings, and parties. The key is figuring out a realistic way to stay keto and be able to enjoy yourself, no matter the situation.

Happy Hour

Happy hours are great opportunities to decompress from hectic workdays, have fun, and connect with friends. And more often than not, happy hours take place at a bar.

On a keto diet, you can absolutely enjoy an occasional alcohol-based drink, as long as you choose low-carb options. My go-tos are dry wines and clear liquors.

DRY RED WINES (3 TO 5 GRAMS OF CARBS PER 5-OUNCE GLASS)

- Cabernet Sauvignon
- Merlot
- Pinot Noir

DRY WHITE WINES (3 TO 5 GRAMS OF CARBS PER 5-OUNCE GLASS)

- Champagne
- Chardonnay
- Pinot Grigio
- Sauvignon Blanc

CLEAR LIQUORS (0 CARBS)

- Brandy
- Cognac
- Gin
- Rum
- Tequila
- Vodka
- Whiskey

MIXERS

- No-sugar-added, naturally flavored sparkling water
- Olive juice (1 ounce typically for dry martinis)
- Seltzer/soda water
- Squeeze of lime or lemon juice
- Water

CKL TIPS

- Avoid tonic water, which is full of sugar.
- Mixed drinks and premade frozen drinks will most likely contain sugar.
- Most beers contain gluten, which can be inflammatory, and are higher in carbs, so opt for wine or liquor when possible.

Work Lunches

Cooking at home and bringing a packed lunch to work is your best bet when it comes to a Clean Keto Lifestyle. But that can get boring and can make you feel a little isolated sometimes. By all means, head out with your coworkers to lunch at a restaurant. Just remember these easy strategies to navigate eating out:

1. **Base your meals around a protein.**
   + Eggs, steak, or salmon are great options. I usually ask the restaurant to grill them or cook them in butter.

2. **Add in healthy fats and veggies to round out your meal.**
   + Salads are great—ask for no croutons, and opt for oil and vinegar in lieu of a sugary salad dressing.
   + Ask for plain steamed veggies (broccoli, asparagus, cauliflower), and then request extra-virgin olive oil, salt, and pepper on the side to season on your own.

3. **Keep starches/grains off your plate to avoid temptation.**
   + If ordering an entrée, substitute a salad or extra veggies for the grain/starch.
   + If ordering a sandwich or a burger, substitute lettuce wraps for the bun.

4. **Be wary of sauces and condiments.**
   + Ketchup, salad dressing, cocktail sauce, barbeque sauce, honey mustard, gravy, and marinara will likely contain sugar and/or flour, so avoid them.
   + Mustard, salsa, guacamole, mayonnaise, béarnaise, and hollandaise should be keto-friendly.
   + If you are unsure about the sauce, ask the server about the ingredients. You can also ask for the sauce on the side so you can control how much is added to your meal.

CKL TIPS

- Look at the menu online before heading to the restaurant so you are prepared. Call the restaurant ahead of time to get any of your questions answered.
- Gluten-free doesn't equal keto, so still be a food detective and ask if there are any added sugars or grains.
- If no entrées on the menu seem to work, feel free to get creative and build a meal with appetizers (oysters and a side salad or a charcuterie plate without the bread and a side of broccoli).

Parties and Gatherings

There is no need to worry about that upcoming party or holiday gathering. By using one or all of the strategies below, you can attend any get-together with no problem at all.

1. Communication is key. If you feel comfortable with the host, give them a quick call well before the party. You will find that most hosts are completely accommodating if they have advance notice. Here are a few ways to broach the topic:

    + Honesty is best. Let the host know that you are on the ketogenic diet and not eating sugar or grains. If that feels uncomfortable, you can take a different approach and tell them you have stomach issues and are trying to avoid eating grains and sugar for a few weeks.

    + Offer to bring something to the party. If they oblige, you can bring a keto-friendly dish to enjoy. Check out the recipe section of this book for tons of great ideas. Adjust the amount of the ingredients based on how many people you need to cook for.

2. Eat before the event. Have a healthy, fat-filled keto meal before arriving. This will keep you in control of your hunger and make it a breeze to pass on the bread basket and sugary dessert.

3. Feel confident in your decision to live a Clean Keto Lifestyle. "No, thank you" is always a perfectly acceptable response. Don't feel pressure to eat something you don't want to or feel you need to make excuses.

4. Enjoy yourself. Dinner parties and holiday gatherings are meant for you to spend quality time with friends and family. Don't overstress or overthink it. Remember, this is only one meal. If you don't eat 100 percent perfect keto, that's okay. Just get back on track with the next meal.

Keto by Cuisine

You are inevitably going to eat out at a restaurant at some point, so here are my strategies on what to order, broken down by cuisine.

DELIS

1. Opt for veggie-filled salads. My favorite is a Cobb salad, or I make my own with spinach, a protein (chicken, ham, shrimp, hard-boiled eggs), healthy fats (olives and avocado), and veggies (onion, broccoli, cucumbers, tomatoes).
2. Pour on the extra-virgin olive oil (and plenty of it!) and vinegar of your choice as the dressing. Avoid any dressing that might have sugar added, including raspberry or balsamic vinaigrette, French, Thousand Island, ranch, or honey mustard.

BURGER JOINTS

1. Choose a burger with the highest quality meat. Grass-fed beef and bison are great choices. Ask for a lettuce wrap in lieu of a bun. If that isn't available, then ask for no bun at all.
2. Choose toppings like tomato, onion, avocado, pickles, bacon, and cheese.
3. When it comes to condiments, avoid ketchup and barbecue sauce, which are full of sugar, and instead go for mustard and mayo.
4. When it comes to sides, pass on the fries and onion rings and instead ask for a side salad or some steamed veggies.

MEXICAN RESTAURANTS

1. Can we say guacamole? This is a great option, but pass on those tortilla chips and ask for crudités instead.
2. Try taco salads and burrito bowls with carnitas, steak, chicken, or shrimp. Swap the rice for greens, eliminate the beans, and feel free to add guacamole, salsa, sour cream, onions, bell peppers, and jalapeños.
3. Fajitas without the tortillas, rice, and beans also work.

1. Skip the rice, and order rolls that are wrapped in cucumber (these are called Naruto rolls).
2. Tuna, salmon, or crab Naruto rolls are great, but stay away from tempura or anything that is battered. Also, make sure to fill the roll with avocado or cream cheese to get your healthy fats in.
3. Bring your own coconut aminos from home (they also sell small packets that you can keep in your purse), rather than using the soy sauce at the restaurant.
4. Other great options are handrolls made without rice and wrapped in seaweed paper, sashimi (raw fish), and miso soup.

Keto with Your Family and Friends

MAKE IT A FAMILY AFFAIR

You can use a Clean Keto Lifestyle to help your family improve their eating habits, as well. Rather than saying, "Mom/Dad is on a diet," and then eating your own separate food, tell your family that you are going to work together to improve everyone's health through better eating. Explain to your kids the importance of brainpower, strong muscles, and energy to work and play, and how what you eat impacts these things.

Get your family involved in the cooking. Give them simple cooking tasks (stirring, seasoning, measuring), and teach them about the ingredients as you go. Let them taste the food and try new things. By getting them personally involved, they will be excited about the food choices in your home, which will help them develop an affinity for healthy foods. Cooking together is also a great bonding experience that gives everyone a chance to talk and enjoy each other's company.

With your family involved, sticking to a Clean Keto Lifestyle will be that much easier!

FIND A SUPPORT SYSTEM

Identify one person who knows how to give you unwavering support (your best friend, a significant other, a parent, or even a coworker). Use this person to hold you accountable and be your biggest cheerleader as you go through this process. Life isn't perfect, and you will ultimately stumble or encounter some challenges. Leverage your support person during these times, and stay the keto course. It is a journey, not a race. The key is to make this a lifestyle.

Another strategy is to identify one person who can work out with you. This can be the same support person or someone else. Exercising is definitely easier and more fun when someone is doing it alongside you. Your workout buddy will also keep you motivated and hold you accountable.

TAKE INITIATIVE WHEN IT COMES TO YOUR SOCIAL GROUP

Going keto doesn't mean that you have to give up your social life. It just requires taking some initiative when it comes to your group of friends. If you are going out to eat, take charge of where the group eats, confirming in advance that there are healthy, keto-friendly choices for you at the restaurant. Or better yet, organize gatherings at someone's house, where you can bring your own keto dishes.

Be open with your friends. Let them know about your new lifestyle, and talk to them about your journey and what changes you are implementing. If they are true friends, they will provide you with encouragement and love. Plus, once they see your amazing results, they are definitely going to be asking you all about how to get the same for themselves. Pay it forward, and pass along your knowledge and words of advice.

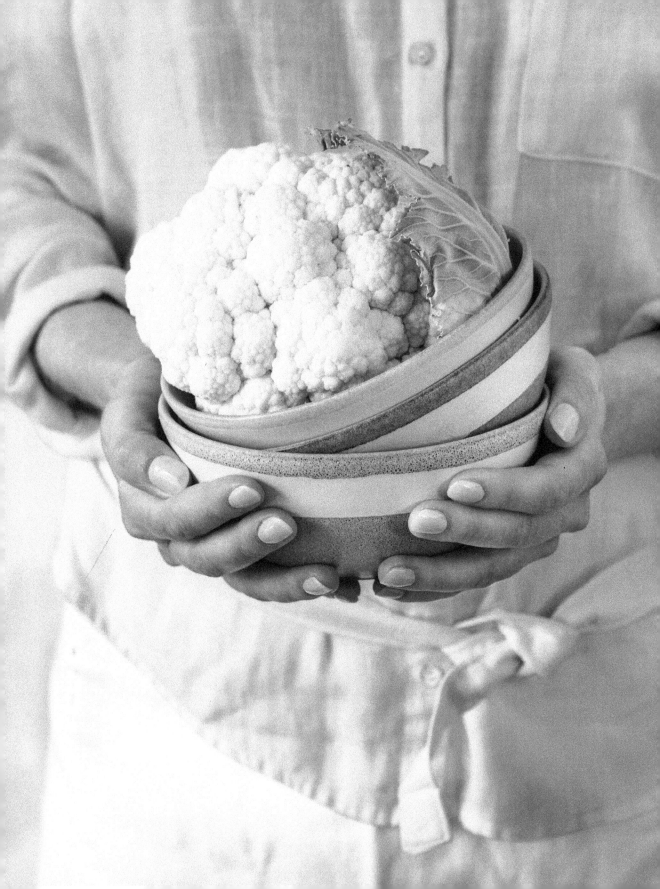

PART TWO

Clean Keto Recipes

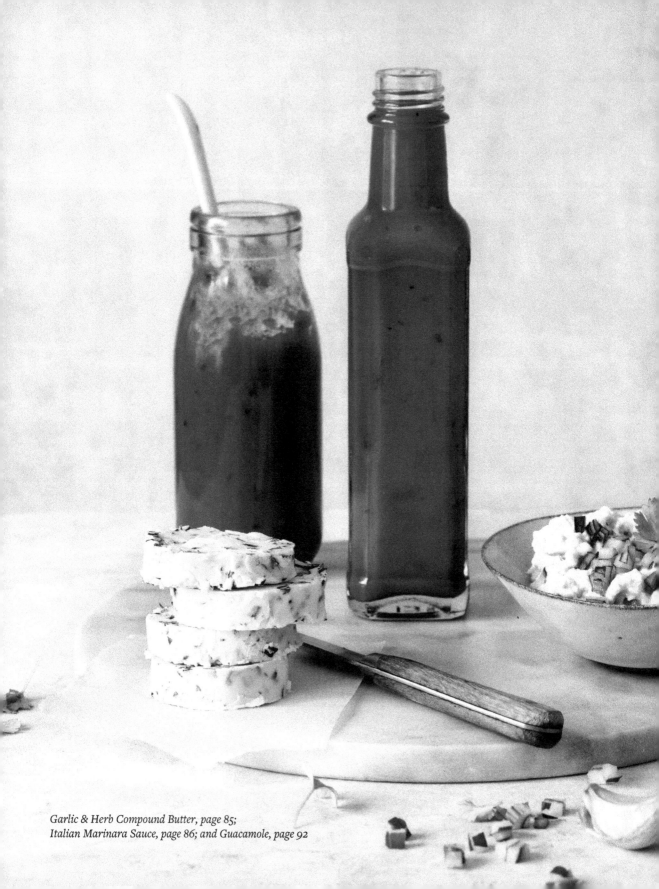

Garlic & Herb Compound Butter, page 85;
Italian Marinara Sauce, page 86; and Guacamole, page 92

6

SEASONINGS, SAUCES, DRESSINGS & DIPS

ITALIAN SEASONING

YIELD: 12 servings (1 tablespoon per serving)

2 tablespoons dried basil

2 tablespoons
dried oregano

2 tablespoons
dried rosemary

2 tablespoons
garlic powder

2 tablespoons dried thyme

2 teaspoons red
pepper flakes

Make dried spices a staple in your kitchen. Not only do they add instant flavor to any dish, but they also last a long time. I love experimenting with spice blends when I cook, and this Italian Seasoning turned out to be the perfect flavor combo for adding to tomato sauces, dressings, and meatballs. Make extra and store it in your pantry for future use.

1. Combine all the spices.
2. Store in a sealed container at room temperature for up to 6 months.

PER SERVING
Macronutrients: Fat 6%; Protein 11%; Carbs 84%
Calories: 11; Total Fat: 0g; Protein: 0g; Total Carbs: 2g; Fiber: 1g; Net Carbs: 1g

RANCH SEASONING

YIELD: *10 servings (1 tablespoon per serving)*

6 tablespoons dried dill

1 tablespoon pink
   Himalayan salt

1 tablespoon freshly ground
   black pepper

1 tablespoon onion powder

1 tablespoon garlic powder

There is no need to spend money on store-bought ranch seasoning packets that contain additives and preservatives that you don't want or need. The combination of herbs and spices in this blend makes the perfect homemade, keto-friendly ranch dressing. Try adding it to any dish that needs a little extra pizzazz.

1. Combine all the spices.

2. Store in a sealed container at room temperature for up to 6 months.

PER SERVING
Macronutrients: Fat 0%; Protein 25%; Carbs 75%
Calories: 12; Total Fat: 0g; Protein: 1g; Total Carbs: 3g; Fiber: 1g; Net Carbs: 2g

TACO SEASONING

YIELD: *8 servings (1 tablespoon per serving)*

4 tablespoons
ground cumin

1 tablespoon garlic powder

1 tablespoon chili powder

1 tablespoon onion powder

2 teaspoons dried oregano

2 teaspoons paprika

Give any meal some Mexican flare with this super easy Taco Seasoning. Mix it into ground beef or rub it onto chicken, steak, or shrimp, and get ready to experience a fiesta in your mouth. It also tastes great mixed into sour cream or melted cheese for a quick dip.

1. Combine all the spices.
2. Store in a sealed container at room temperature for up to 6 months.

PER SERVING
Macronutrients: Fat 31%; Protein 14%; Carbs 55%
Calories: 29; Total Fat: 1g; Protein: 1g; Total Carbs: 4g; Fiber: 1g; Net Carbs: 3g

GARLIC & HERB COMPOUND BUTTER

YIELD: *4 servings (1 tablespoon per serving)*

4 tablespoons (½ stick) grass-fed butter, at room temperature

¾ teaspoon freshly squeezed lemon juice

1 garlic clove, minced

1 teaspoon finely chopped fresh parsley

1 teaspoon finely chopped fresh herbs (such as basil, oregano, or rosemary)

It's amazing what adding garlic and fresh herbs to butter can do. Melt it on steak, seafood, eggs, or cooked veggies, and an ordinary meal becomes good enough for company.

1. Combine all of the ingredients in a bowl and mix thoroughly.
2. Season with salt and freshly ground black pepper to taste.
3. Place the mixture on a piece of plastic wrap, and roll it into a log.
4. Twist the ends to seal well.
5. Refrigerate for at least 1 hour before using.

CKL TIP: Store the butter for up to 5 days in the refrigerator or up to 6 months in the freezer. If freezing, cut the log into individual rounds and freeze them separately to make it easy to use whenever you like.

PER SERVING
Macronutrients: Fat 100%; Protein 0%; Carbs 0%
Calories: 108; Total Fat: 12g; Protein: 0g; Total Carbs: 0g; Fiber: 0g; Net Carbs: 0g

ITALIAN MARINARA SAUCE

YIELD: *3 servings (½ cup per serving)*

1 tablespoon avocado oil

4 garlic cloves, minced

1 (12-ounce) can plain
  tomato sauce

2 tablespoons Italian
  Seasoning (page 82)

Enjoy the classic taste of a traditional marinara sauce without all the added sugar that you find in most store brands. This sauce is perfect spooned over a big bowl of zucchini noodles and meatballs. Double or triple the batch and store it in the freezer, and you'll have the base for a few easy meals in the future.

1. Place the oil and garlic in a saucepan over medium heat.

2. Sauté until the garlic starts to sizzle, about 1 minute.

3. Pour the tomato sauce into the saucepan and add the Italian Seasoning.

4. Stir to combine everything, and bring to a light boil.

5. Reduce the heat to low, and simmer for about 20 minutes. Stir occasionally.

6. Remove from the heat, let cool, and store in a sealed container.

PER SERVING
Macronutrients: Fat 79%; Protein 0%; Carbs 21%
Calories: 57; Total Fat: 5g; Protein: 0g; Total Carbs: 3g; Fiber: 1g; Net Carbs: 2g

BASIL PESTO

YIELD: *8 servings (2 tablespoons per serving)*

3 cups fresh basil leaves

2 garlic cloves, halved

¼ cup raw whole almonds

¼ teaspoon pink
    Himalayan salt

¼ cup extra-virgin olive oil

A secret weapon for livening up any keto dish, this pesto is also the perfect recipe to make if you want to use up all that fresh basil growing in your garden. Add it to scrambled eggs, roasted fish, steamed veggies, or any Italian dish to achieve that next level of flavor.

1. Place the basil leaves, garlic, almonds, and salt in a blender or food processor.

2. Blend continuously until the ingredients start to break down, about 20 seconds.

3. Slowly pour in the oil, and continue to blend until the oil is fully incorporated.

CKL TIP: Basil Pesto can be stored in a sealed container in the refrigerator for up to 7 days. You can also freeze the pesto in ice cube trays, transfer them to a zip-top bag, and store them in the freezer for up to 6 months.

PER SERVING
Macronutrients: Fat 90%; Protein 5%; Carbs 5%
Calories: 80; Total Fat: 8g; Protein: 1g; Total Carbs: 1g; Fiber: 1g; Net Carbs: 0g

CHIMICHURRI

YIELD: *8 servings (2 tablespoons per serving)*

1 cup fresh cilantro

2 cups fresh parsley

¼ cup red wine vinegar

3 garlic cloves, halved

½ teaspoon ground cumin

½ teaspoon red
pepper flakes

¼ teaspoon pink
Himalayan salt

¼ cup extra-virgin olive oil

Beautifully green and packing a solid punch of flavor, chimichurri is a sauce originating from Argentina, and it's a great complement to any cooked meat or seafood. I love drizzling it over a perfectly grilled flank steak.

1. Place the cilantro, parsley, vinegar, garlic, cumin, red pepper flakes, and salt in a blender or food processor.

2. Blend continuously until the ingredients start to break down, about 20 seconds.

3. Slowly pour in the oil, and continue to blend until the oil is fully incorporated.

PER SERVING

Macronutrients: Fat 82%; Protein 6%; Carbs 12%
Calories: 66; Total Fat: 6g; Protein: 1g; Total Carbs: 2g; Fiber: 1g; Net Carbs: 1g

SIMPLE BALSAMIC VINAIGRETTE

YIELD: *2 servings (2 tablespoons per serving)*

1½ tablespoons
  balsamic vinegar

½ tablespoon
  Dijon mustard

1 garlic clove, minced

2 tablespoons extra-virgin
  olive oil

This salad dressing is so simple to make, and the flavor is the perfect combination of tangy and tasty. I love pouring it over salads, roasted veggies, and baked chicken thighs. I make a large batch on the weekend and store it in the refrigerator to use throughout the week.

1. In a small bowl, whisk the vinegar, Dijon mustard, and garlic together until well combined.
2. Slowly drizzle in the oil, and whisk until it emulsifies and thickens.
3. Season with salt and freshly ground black pepper to taste.

PER SERVING
Macronutrients: Fat 91%; Protein 0%; Carbs 9%
Calories: 138; Total Fat: 14g; Protein: 0g; Total Carbs: 3g; Fiber: 0g; Net Carbs: 3g

ITALIAN VINAIGRETTE

YIELD: *2 servings (2 tablespoons per serving)*

2 tablespoons red
   wine vinegar

1 garlic clove, minced

1 teaspoon Italian
   Seasoning (page 82)

2 tablespoons extra-virgin
   olive oil

My husband is Italian and can't get enough of this dressing. The secret is the homemade seasoning blend that is chock-full of flavorful herbs and spices that are native to Italy. It tastes great paired with fresh greens and crisp vegetables for an incredible salad.

1. In a small bowl, whisk the vinegar, garlic, and Italian Seasoning together until well combined.

2. Slowly drizzle in the oil, and whisk until it emulsifies and thickens.

3. Season with salt and freshly ground black pepper to taste.

PER SERVING
Macronutrients: Fat 97%; Protein 0%; Carbs 3%
Calories: 130; Total Fat: 14g; Protein: 0g; Total Carbs: 1g; Fiber: 0g; Net Carbs: 1g

KETO RANCH

YIELD: *8 servings (¼ cup per serving)*

2 eggs, ideally at room temperature

4 tablespoons red wine vinegar

2 tablespoons Ranch Seasoning (page 83)

1⅓ cups avocado oil

4 tablespoons unsweetened full-fat coconut milk

Keto Ranch can easily be made at home in just a few minutes and tastes just as good as, if not better than, store-bought ranch dressings, which have added sugars and refined oils. This versatile recipe can be used as a salad dressing or dip, and will soon become a staple in your refrigerator.

1. Put the eggs, vinegar, and Ranch Seasoning in a blender or food processor.
2. Pulse a few times to combine the ingredients.
3. Start the blender or food processor and slowly pour in the oil through the top.
4. Once all of the oil has been incorporated, add the coconut milk and blend or pulse for a few more seconds.

PER SERVING
Macronutrients: Fat 96%; Protein 3%; Carbs 1%
Calories: 358; Total Fat: 38g; Protein: 2g; Total Carbs: 1g; Fiber: 0g; Net Carbs: 1g

GUACAMOLE

YIELD: *2 servings (½ cup per serving)*

1 avocado, halved, pitted, and peeled

1 teaspoon lime juice

¼ medium red onion, diced

¼ tablespoon ground cumin

¼ tablespoon garlic powder

1 teaspoon minced fresh cilantro (optional)

Holy guacamole! Here is my spin on a classic: I add cumin and garlic powder for some additional spice. Whether you eat it with a spoon, use it as a dip, or pile it high on a taco salad, you can't go wrong with guacamole.

1. Place the avocado halves in a medium bowl.
2. With a fork, mash the avocado to your preferred consistency.
3. Add the remaining ingredients to the mashed avocado, and mix well.
4. Season with salt to taste.

PER SERVING

Macronutrients: Fat 71%; Protein 5%; Carbs 24%
Calories: 165; Total Fat: 13g; Protein: 2g; Total Carbs: 10g; Fiber: 6g; Net Carbs: 4g

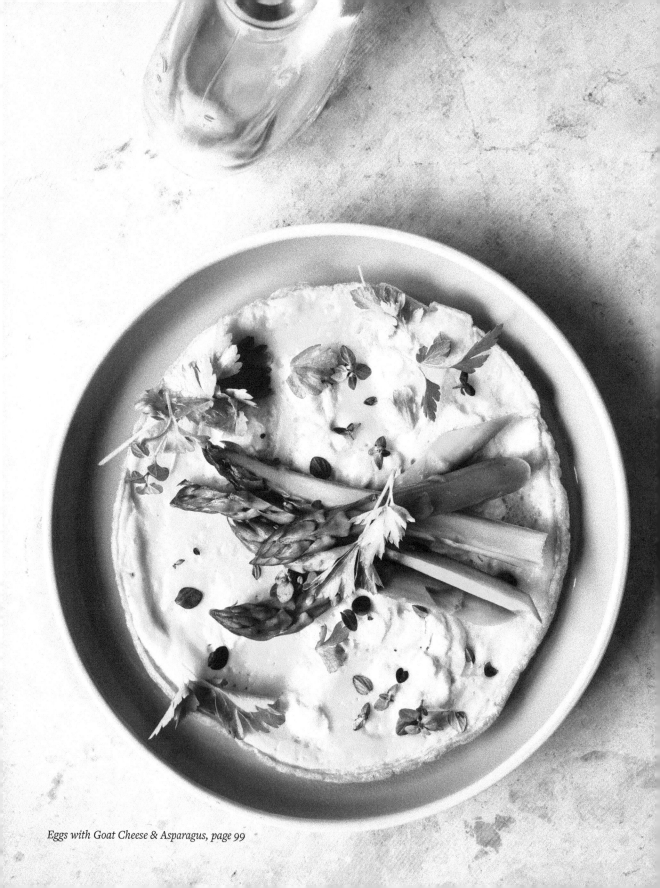

Eggs with Goat Cheese & Asparagus, page 99

BREAKFAST DISHES

TURKEY EGG SCRAMBLE

YIELD: *1 serving*

1 teaspoon avocado oil

¼ medium red onion, diced

¼ red bell pepper, diced

2 garlic cloves, minced

4 ounces ground turkey

¼ teaspoon chili powder

2 eggs

¼ cup fresh spinach

On Saturday mornings, my husband always makes an egg scramble with whatever he finds in the refrigerator. He is very creative in the kitchen, and I never know what flavor combo he is going to create. This one was a winner, hands-down!

1. In a skillet, heat the oil over medium heat.
2. Add the onion, bell pepper, and garlic and sauté for 5 to 7 minutes until soft.
3. Add the turkey, then season with the chili powder and salt and freshly ground black pepper to taste.
4. Continue to cook until the turkey begins to brown.
5. In a small bowl, beat the eggs, and pour them into the skillet over the turkey and vegetables.
6. Layer the spinach on top of the eggs, stir to combine, and continue to cook until the eggs are set.

CKL TIP: Throw any leftover vegetables or herbs into this scramble. It's a great way to clean out your refrigerator at the end of the week!

PER SERVING
Macronutrients: Fat 56%; Protein 35%; Carbs 9%
Calories: 367; Total Fat: 23g; Protein: 32g; Total Carbs: 8g; Fiber: 2g; Net Carbs: 6g

EGGS & BACON

YIELD: *1 serving*

2 bacon slices

1 tablespoon avocado oil

2 eggs

Is there anything better than the smell of bacon cooking in a skillet? I'm so glad eggs and bacon is a keto classic. I've fried the eggs here, but feel free to cook your eggs however you like—scrambled, sunny-side up, over medium, boiled, or poached.

1. In a small skillet, cook the bacon over medium heat until crispy and brown.

2. Transfer the bacon to a paper towel–lined plate.

3. Pour the excess bacon grease from the skillet into a glass jar to use in another recipe (see CKL tip).

4. Into the same skillet over medium heat, pour the oil.

5. Add the eggs, and fry until thoroughly cooked.

CKL TIP: Save the bacon grease to use for sautéing and roasting. Cooking with bacon grease adds a whole new layer of flavor.

PER SERVING

Macronutrients: Fat 77%; Protein 22%; Carbs 1%
Calories: 455; Total Fat: 39g; Protein: 25g; Total Carbs: 1g; Fiber: 0g; Net Carbs: 1g

PROSCIUTTO EGG CUPS

YIELD: *1 serving (2 cups per person)*

2 eggs

½ cup chopped
  fresh spinach

1 scallion, finely sliced

1 tablespoon unsweetened
  full-fat coconut milk

1 teaspoon coconut oil

2 prosciutto slices,
  folded in half

I love making these egg cups when I have guests over because I can cook twelve of them at a time in a muffin pan. If you do this, be sure to multiply the ingredients by six. They also look beautiful on a platter. Serve with a colorful salad for the ultimate keto brunch.

1. Preheat the oven to 350°F.

2. In a small bowl, beat the eggs, add the spinach and scallion, and mix together.

3. Mix in the coconut milk, and season with a little salt and freshly ground black pepper.

4. Grease two cups of a muffin tin with the coconut oil, and line each cup with a folded slice of prosciutto.

5. Fill each cup about two-thirds full with the egg mixture.

6. Bake for 30 minutes, until the eggs are fully cooked.

PER SERVING
Macronutrients: Fat 66%; Protein 30%; Carbs 4%
Calories: 302; Total Fat: 22g; Protein: 23g; Total Carbs: 3g; Fiber: 1g; Net Carbs: 2g

PREP TIME: 5 minutes
COOK TIME: 15 minutes

EGGS WITH GOAT CHEESE & ASPARAGUS

YIELD: *1 serving*

3 asparagus spears, woody ends removed

2 eggs

1 tablespoon avocado oil

1 tablespoon goat cheese

1 teaspoon extra-virgin olive oil, for drizzling

A few leaves of cilantro or other fresh herbs (optional)

This dish is inspired by an unforgettable breakfast that I had in Paris. The goat cheese combined with the eggs creates the creamiest texture. Add some fresh herbs to the eggs if you like, and drizzle the asparagus with a good quality extra-virgin olive oil.

1. In a small skillet, heat 2 tablespoons of water over medium-high heat.
2. Add the asparagus, cover, and steam until the water has evaporated and the asparagus is tender.
3. Place the asparagus on a plate, slice them in half lengthwise, and set aside.
4. In a small bowl, beat the eggs.
5. Pour out any water left in the skillet. Add the avocado oil, and heat over medium heat.
6. Add the eggs and goat cheese to the skillet, and season with salt and freshly ground black pepper.
7. Cook until the eggs are set and the goat cheese is melted.
8. Serve alongside the asparagus with the olive oil drizzled over top. Garnish with cilantro or fresh herbs of your choice.

PER SERVING
Macronutrients: Fat 78%; Protein 17%; Carbs 5%
Calories: 334; Total Fat: 29g; Protein: 14g; Total Carbs: 4g; Fiber: 2g; Net Carbs: 2g

ITALIAN OMELET

YIELD: *1 serving*

1 tablespoon grass-fed
butter or ghee

1 prosciutto slice, chopped

4 cherry tomatoes, halved

¼ cup fresh spinach

2 eggs

1 teaspoon Italian
Seasoning (page 82)

1 tablespoon Basil Pesto
(page 87)

I absolutely love omelets, and this Italian version is by far my favorite. The Italian Seasoning and the Basil Pesto add so much bright flavor, while the prosciutto adds a salty richness to the dish.

1. In a skillet, melt the butter over medium heat.
2. Add the prosciutto, tomatoes, and spinach, and cook for 2 minutes.
3. In a small bowl, beat the eggs and the Italian Seasoning together.
4. Pour the eggs into the skillet over the prosciutto, tomatoes, and spinach, and move the pan around to spread them out evenly.
5. When the omelet begins to firm up but still has a little raw egg on top, ease around the edges of the omelet with a spatula and then fold it in half.
6. Let it cook for a few more minutes, checking often to see when the bottom of the omelet looks golden brown.
7. When golden brown, turn off the heat and slide the omelet onto a plate.
8. Drizzle with the Basil Pesto.

PER SERVING
Macronutrients: Fat 72%; Protein 23%; Carbs 5%
Calories: 365; Total Fat: 29g; Protein: 21g; Total Carbs: 5g; Fiber: 1g; Net Carbs: 4g

OVERNIGHT CHIA PUDDING

YIELD: *1 serving*

2 tablespoons chia seeds

1 cup unsweetened full-fat
coconut milk

½ teaspoon vanilla extract

½ teaspoon stevia
or 4 drops liquid
stevia extract

Overnight Chia Pudding is a perfect make-ahead, on-the-go keto breakfast. I usually make multiple servings at a time in separate mason jars, so they are ready in the refrigerator and I can grab one before running out the door. Eat it plain or top it with a small handful of berries.

1. In a mason jar, mix together the chia seeds, milk, vanilla, and stevia.

2. Put the lid on the jar and shake to combine everything.

3. Once the chia pudding mixture is well combined, put the jar in the refrigerator for at least 2 hours.

PER SERVING
Macronutrients: Fat 86%; Protein 5%; Carbs 9%
Calories: 588; Total Fat: 57g; Protein: 9g; Total Carbs: 14g; Fiber: 10g; Net Carbs: 4g

COCONUT GRANOLA

YIELD: *3 servings (½ cup per serving)*

- ½ cup chopped raw macadamia nuts
- ½ cup sliced raw almonds
- ¼ cup cacao nibs
- 2 tablespoons unsweetened coconut flakes
- 1 teaspoon vanilla extract
- 1 teaspoon ground cinnamon
- ¼ teaspoon pink Himalayan salt
- 2 tablespoons melted coconut oil

Coconut Granola is my clean, keto–friendly version of those store-bought cereals that are full of grains and tons of added sugar. The sweetness in this granola comes from the coconut. Serve it as a cereal replacement or as a crunchy topping for full-fat plain yogurt.

1. Preheat the oven to 325°F. Line a baking sheet with parchment paper.

2. In a food processor or with a knife, chop the macadamia nuts into smaller pieces.

3. Place the macadamia nuts, almonds, cacao nibs, coconut, vanilla, cinnamon, and salt in a medium bowl, add the coconut oil, and mix well.

4. Pour the granola onto the baking sheet, and spread it out in an even layer.

5. Bake for 15 to 20 minutes or just until it is fragrant and toasted on the bottom. The mixture can burn easily, so keep an eye on it and stir frequently.

6. Let it cool completely, and serve with 1 cup of almond milk or plain Greek yogurt.

CKL TIP: Double or triple this recipe, and store the extra in a sealed container.

PER SERVING
Macronutrients: Fat 85%; Protein 7%; Carbs 8%
Calories: 433; Total Fat: 43g; Protein: 8g; Total Carbs: 12g; Fiber: 8g; Net Carbs: 4g

GREEN SMOOTHIE

YIELD: *1 serving*

½ avocado, pitted and peeled

½ cup unsweetened full-fat coconut milk

½ cup cold water

1 teaspoon vanilla extract

1 tablespoon MCT oil

½ teaspoon stevia *or* 4 drops liquid stevia extract

1 cup fresh spinach

A few ice cubes (optional)

When I first start working with my clients, we always review what they are eating each day. More often than not, they start their day with a smoothie full of bananas, apples, and other sugary fruits. These fruit-based smoothies are doing more harm than good by spiking your blood sugar ("glu-coaster" time!). Instead, try my Green Smoothie for a healthier, keto-friendly version.

1. In the order listed, place all the ingredients, except the ice, in a blender.

2. Add ice (if using), and blend until smooth.

PER SERVING
Macronutrients: Fat 86%; Protein 4%; Carbs 10%
Calories: 504; Total Fat: 48g; Protein: 5g; Total Carbs: 13g; Fiber: 9g; Net Carbs: 4g

BERRY CHEESECAKE SMOOTHIE

YIELD: *1 serving*

½ cup unsweetened
full-fat coconut milk

½ cup cold water

1 tablespoon MCT oil

¼ cup full-fat
cream cheese

½ teaspoon stevia
or 4 drops liquid
stevia extract

¼ cup blueberries

A few ice cubes (optional)

Here is a keto smoothie that has become a client favorite. The cream cheese provides a creamy, milkshake-like consistency. You will love starting your day with this balanced drink designed to keep you satiated throughout the morning.

1. In the order listed, place all the ingredients, except the ice, in a blender.

2. Add ice (if using), and blend until smooth.

PER SERVING
Macronutrients: Fat 86%; Protein 5%; Carbs 9%
Calories: 575; Total Fat: 55g; Protein: 7g; Total Carbs: 13g; Fiber: 4g; Net Carbs: 9g

CHOCOLATE PROTEIN SHAKE

YIELD: *1 serving*

1 cup unsweetened full-fat coconut milk

1 scoop collagen powder

1 teaspoon cacao powder

1 tablespoon MCT oil

1 cup fresh spinach

½ teaspoon stevia *or* 4 drops liquid stevia extract

A few ice cubes (optional)

I've designed this Chocolate Protein Shake to keep you energized all morning long. In addition to the healthy fats, this smoothie also includes collagen powder, which is great for your skin, hair, and joints.

1. In the order listed, place all the ingredients, except the ice, in a blender.

2. Add ice (if using), and blend until smooth.

PER SERVING

Macronutrients: Fat 78%; Protein 12%; Carbs 10%
Calories: 631; Total Fat: 55g; Protein: 19g; Total Carbs: 15g; Fiber: 8g; Net Carbs: 7g

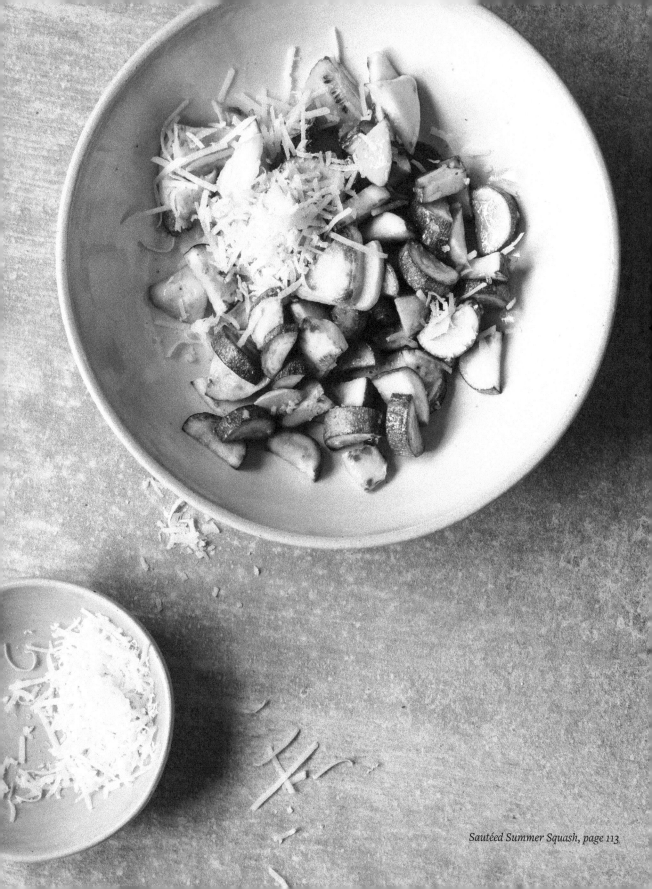

Sautéed Summer Squash, page 113

8

SIDES & SNACKS

ROASTED BROCCOLI

YIELD: *1 serving*

1½ cups broccoli florets

2 tablespoons avocado oil

2 garlic cloves, thinly sliced

Juice of ½ lemon

2 tablespoons raw
   sliced almonds

1 teaspoon freshly grated
   Parmesan cheese
   (optional)

Broccoli is anything but boring in this simple-to-prepare recipe. The lemon juice adds a kick of freshness, and the almonds add a great crunch. As a side dish, it pairs perfectly with any meat or seafood.

1. Preheat the oven to 425°F; line a baking sheet with parchment paper.

2. In a large bowl, toss the broccoli, oil, and garlic until well combined.

3. Season with salt and freshly ground black pepper.

4. Spread the broccoli evenly on the prepared baking sheet, drizzling any excess oil on top, and put the baking sheet in the oven.

5. After 15 minutes, drizzle the lemon juice over the broccoli and top with the almonds and cheese (if using).

6. Continue to bake for an additional 5 to 10 minutes, until the florets are crispy and caramelized.

PER SERVING
Macronutrients: Fat 52%; Protein 15%; Carbs 33%
Calories: 192; Total Fat: 10g; Protein: 7g; Total Carbs: 16g; Fiber: 7g; Net Carbs: 9g

CAULIFLOWER MASH

YIELD: *1 serving*

½ head cauliflower, cut into small florets (about 1½ cups)

1 tablespoon extra-virgin olive oil

1 tablespoon grass-fed butter or ghee

If you haven't tried cauliflower mash yet, be prepared to have your mind blown. Master this basic recipe, and then experiment by adding fresh herbs, dried spices, or heavy cream. My favorite addition is grated horseradish.

1. Bring a large pot of water to a boil over high heat.
2. Add the cauliflower florets and cook until really tender, 8 to 10 minutes.
3. Remove from the heat, strain, and let cool slightly.
4. Transfer the cauliflower to the bowl of a blender or food processor.
5. Add the oil and butter, and blend until smooth and creamy, stopping a few times to scrape down the sides of the blender or food processor bowl.
6. Season to taste with salt and freshly ground black pepper.
7. Serve immediately.

CKL TIP: Top with a dollop of Garlic & Herb Compound Butter (page 85).

PER SERVING
Macronutrients: Fat 85%; Protein 4%; Carbs 11%
Calories: 274; Total Fat: 26g; Protein: 3g; Total Carbs: 7g; Fiber: 3g; Net Carbs: 4g

CRISPY BRUSSELS SPROUTS

YIELD: *1 serving*

⅓ pound Brussels sprouts, trimmed and thinly sliced (about 1½ cups)

2 garlic cloves, minced

2 tablespoons avocado oil

Juice of ½ lemon

1 teaspoon freshly grated Parmesan cheese (optional)

Talk about a comeback: Brussels sprouts went from being one of the most avoided veggies out there to being a mainstay on restaurant menus everywhere. Here is my favorite way to eat them. Warning—these are extremely addicting!

1. Preheat the oven to 400°F; line a baking sheet with parchment paper.
2. Place the thinly sliced Brussels sprouts and garlic on the lined baking sheet.
3. Cover well with the oil, and season with salt and freshly ground black pepper to taste.
4. Using your hands, mix all the ingredients together, then spread everything out in one even layer.
5. Roast in the oven for 20 to 25 minutes, stirring every 8 to 10 minutes, until the Brussels sprouts are tender.
6. Transfer to a bowl, drizzle with the lemon juice, and stir to combine. Sprinkle with the cheese (if using).

PER SERVING
Macronutrients: Fat 68%; Protein 8%; Carbs 24%
Calories: 385; Total Fat: 29g; Protein: 8g; Total Carbs: 23g; Fiber: 10g; Net Carbs: 13g

MEXICAN CAULIFLOWER RICE

YIELD: *1 serving*

½ head cauliflower,
   cut into small florets
   (about 1½ cups)

1 tablespoon avocado oil

1 garlic clove, minced

¼ cup tomato sauce

¼ cup water or broth

1 teaspoon onion powder

½ teaspoon ground cumin

Juice of ½ lime

1 tablespoon minced fresh
   cilantro (optional)

Cauliflower makes a perfect substitution for rice, and it couldn't be simpler to make. I've added cumin, cilantro, and a little lime juice to give this side dish a Mexican twist. Use it as a base for a taco salad, or serve it alongside fajitas.

1. Place the cauliflower florets in a food processor, and process until the mixture resembles rice.

2. In a large skillet, heat the oil over medium heat.

3. Add the cauliflower "rice" and garlic to the skillet, and cook for 5 minutes.

4. Stir in the tomato sauce, water, onion powder, and cumin. Season with salt and freshly ground black pepper to taste.

5. Cover and cook for 5 to 10 more minutes, until tender.

6. Uncover, toss with the lime juice, and garnish with the cilantro (if using).

PER SERVING
Macronutrients: Fat 62%; Protein 7%; Carbs 31%
Calories: 219; Total Fat: 15g; Protein: 4g; Total Carbs: 17g; Fiber: 5g; Net Carbs: 12g

ROASTED MUSHROOMS

YIELD: *1 serving*

1 (8-ounce) package sliced
cremini mushrooms

1 tablespoon Garlic &
Herb Compound Butter
(page 85)

Roasted mushrooms are so easy to prepare, and they are a classic accompaniment to a beautifully prepared steak. If you are dairy intolerant, swap out the compound butter for avocado oil and minced garlic—it will taste just as good, I promise.

1. Preheat the oven to 375°F; line a baking sheet with parchment paper.

2. In a bowl, combine the mushrooms and the compound butter. Season with salt and freshly ground black pepper to taste.

3. Place the mushrooms in a single layer on the lined baking sheet.

4. Bake for 12 to 15 minutes, tossing occasionally, until browned and tender.

PER SERVING
Macronutrients: Fat 64%; Protein 14%; Carbs 22%
Calories: 168; Total Fat: 12g; Protein: 6g; Total Carbs: 9g; Fiber: 2g; Net Carbs: 7g

SAUTÉED SUMMER SQUASH

YIELD: *1 serving*

1 tablespoon avocado oil

½ zucchini, cut into
half-moons

½ yellow summer squash,
cut into half-moons

1 teaspoon freshly grated
Parmesan cheese
(optional)

I am a huge fan of summer squash—especially because of its versatility. You can eat it sliced, chopped, or spiralized. Plus, its flavor is mild enough that you can mix and match seasonings. Feel free to add different spices to this dish to make it your own.

1. In a large skillet, heat the oil over medium heat.

2. Add the zucchini and yellow squash in as even a layer as possible. It should sizzle as it hits the skillet. Sprinkle with salt and freshly ground black pepper.

3. Let the squash sit without stirring or moving for 2 minutes so it can get nice and golden.

4. After 2 minutes, give it a good stir, and then let it continue to cook for an additional 5 minutes, stirring occasionally, until the squash is tender.

5. Transfer to a bowl and sprinkle with the cheese (if using).

PER SERVING
Macronutrients: Fat 78%; Protein 5%; Carbs 17%
Calories: 162; Total Fat: 14g; Protein: 2g; Total Carbs: 7g; Fiber: 2g; Net Carbs: 5g

GARLICKY KALE

YIELD: *1 serving*

1 tablespoon avocado oil

4 garlic cloves, sliced

½ bunch lacinato kale, stemmed

¼ cup water or chicken broth

Kale is known more for its incredible nutritional profile than for its taste, but this dish is going to prove to you how delicious kale can really be. The amount of kale might seem like a lot, but it will reduce in size as it cooks.

1. In a large skillet, heat the oil over medium heat.

2. Add the garlic and let it cook for 1 to 2 minutes, until it starts to sizzle.

3. Add the kale and toss with tongs to coat it fully in the oil.

4. Add the water, season with salt and freshly ground black pepper, and reduce the heat to low.

5. Cook for 20 minutes, until the kale is tender and most of the liquid has evaporated.

PER SERVING
Macronutrients: Fat 63%; Protein 10%; Carbs 27%
Calories: 192; Total Fat: 14g; Protein: 4g; Total Carbs: 13g; Fiber: 2g; Net Carbs: 11g

CREAMED SPINACH

YIELD: *1 serving*

1 tablespoon avocado oil

1 tablespoon grass-fed butter or ghee

¼ medium white onion, diced

2 garlic cloves, minced

1 tablespoon cream cheese

1 teaspoon freshly grated Parmesan cheese

6 cups fresh spinach

This recipe rivals any version that you would find at a fancy steakhouse. It is rich, flavorful, and totally keto. Serve it straight from the skillet, or transfer it to an oven-safe dish, sprinkle it with some additional Parmesan, and bake until the cheese is melted.

1. In a skillet, heat the oil and butter over medium heat.

2. Add the onion and garlic, and sauté for 5 to 7 minutes or until the onion is soft.

3. Whisk in the cream cheese and Parmesan cheese until they are completely melted.

4. Fold in the spinach until evenly combined (add a little water if the mixture seems dry).

5. Season with salt and freshly ground black pepper to taste.

6. Cook for 5 minutes or until the spinach is fully wilted.

PER SERVING
Macronutrients: Fat 77%; Protein 10%; Carbs 13%
Calories: 363; Total Fat: 31g; Protein: 9g; Total Carbs: 12g; Fiber: 5g; Net Carbs: 7g

ASIAN SPICED CUCUMBERS

YIELD: *1 serving*

½ cucumber, peeled
and diced

1 scallion, finely sliced

½ tablespoon sesame oil

½ tablespoon rice vinegar

½ teaspoon sesame seeds

¼ teaspoon red
pepper flakes

Here is a fun, Asian-inspired spin on cucumbers. It makes a
new and interesting side dish to bring to your next family
gathering or to serve at a dinner party. Make it ahead of
time, and leave it in the refrigerator for a bit to allow the
flavors to come alive.

1. Put the diced cucumber in a small bowl.
2. Add the scallion, sesame oil, rice vinegar, sesame seeds,
   and red pepper flakes; stir to combine.
3. Cover the bowl with plastic wrap, and refrigerate for at
   least 30 minutes or up to 24 hours.

PER SERVING
Macronutrients: Fat 67%; Protein 7%; Carbs 26%
Calories: 108; Total Fat: 8g; Protein: 2g; Total Carbs: 7g; Fiber: 2g; Net Carbs: 5g

SOUTHERN GREEN BEANS

YIELD: *1 serving*

½ pound green
    beans, trimmed

¼ cup chopped pecans

1 tablespoon grass-fed
    butter or ghee

2 garlic cloves, minced

If you haven't tried the magical combination of green beans, pecans, garlic, and butter, you are missing out! This is one of my most requested dishes, and it comes together in a flash. Simply combine the ingredients and bake.

1. Preheat the oven to 450°F; line a baking sheet with parchment paper.

2. In a medium bowl, mix together the green beans, pecans, butter, and garlic.

3. Spread out the mixture in one even layer on the prepared baking sheet.

4. Roast in the oven for 20 to 25 minutes.

PER SERVING
Macronutrients: Fat 61%; Protein 8%; Carbs 31%
Calories: 249; Total Fat: 17g; Protein: 5g; Total Carbs: 19g; Fiber: 10g; Net Carbs: 9g

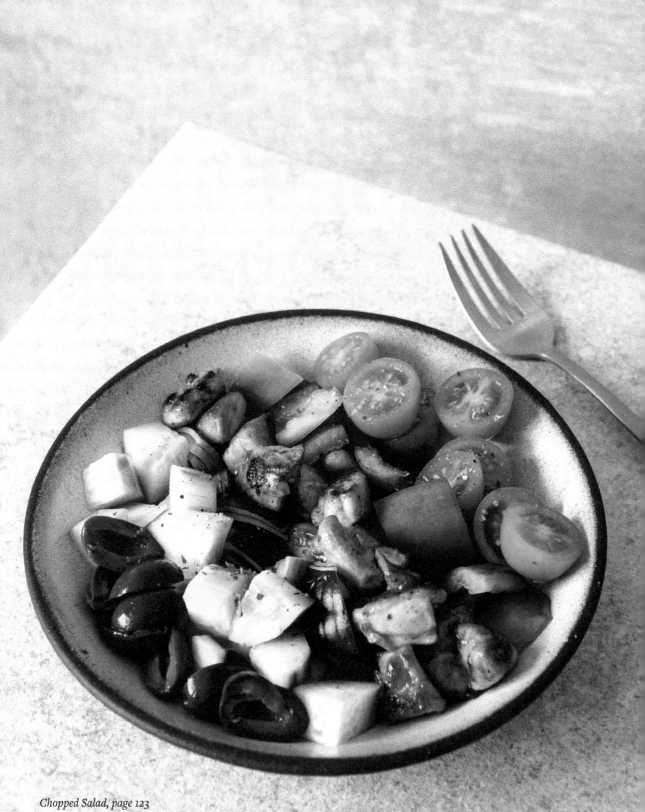

Chopped Salad, page 123

9

SOUPS & SALADS

SHRIMP & AVOCADO SALAD

YIELD: *1 serving*

2 cups mixed greens

4 cherry tomatoes, halved

1 scallion, finely sliced

1 avocado, pitted, peeled,
   and diced

6 ounces cooked shrimp

2 tablespoons Simple
   Balsamic Vinaigrette
   (page 89)

Combining two of my favorite foods—shrimp and avocado—this salad has become a go-to of mine, since it's so easy to prepare. If you cook the shrimp in advance and let them chill in the refrigerator, you can assemble the rest of the salad in a few short minutes.

1. Place the mixed greens in a medium bowl.

2. Top with the tomatoes, scallion, avocado, and shrimp.

3. Drizzle the Simple Balsamic Vinaigrette onto the salad.

PER SERVING
Macronutrients: Fat 56%; Protein 27%; Carbs 17%
Calories: 674; Total Fat: 42g; Protein: 45g; Total Carbs: 29g; Fiber: 16g;
   Net Carbs: 13g

ITALIAN TUNA SALAD

YIELD: *1 serving*

1 (5-ounce) can tuna packed in olive oil

4 cherry tomatoes, halved

¼ medium red onion, cut into half-inch pieces

4 kalamata olives, pitted and halved

2 tablespoons Italian Vinaigrette (page 90)

You will love this new take on regular tuna salad. By swapping the mayonnaise for Italian Vinaigrette, you get a completely different flavor profile. This salad tastes incredibly fresh and is perfect on a hot summer day.

1. Combine all the ingredients in a bowl; mix gently.

2. Season with salt and freshly ground black pepper to taste.

PER SERVING
Macronutrients: Fat 63%; Protein 27%; Carbs 10%
Calories: 430; Total Fat: 28g; Protein: 39g; Total Carbs: 10g; Fiber: 2g; Net Carbs: 8g

CHEF SALAD

YIELD: *1 serving*

2 cups mixed greens

4 cherry tomatoes, halved

1 scallion, finely sliced

1 hard-boiled egg, peeled
and quartered

½ avocado, pitted, peeled,
and diced

1 cooked boneless chicken
thigh, diced

2 tablespoons Simple
Balsamic Vinaigrette
(page 89)

Chef salads are one of my weekly staples on the ketogenic diet. They are versatile, delicious, filling, and they make a perfect lunch that can easily be prepped ahead of time. Swap out the chicken for bacon or the avocado for olives if you want to try something a little different.

1. Place the mixed greens on a plate or in a large bowl.

2. Top with the tomatoes, scallion, egg, avocado, and chicken.

3. Drizzle with the Simple Balsamic Vinaigrette.

CKL TIP: My method for hard-boiling eggs: Place the eggs in a small pot or saucepan, and add cold water to cover the eggs by a few inches. On a stovetop over high heat, bring the water to a gentle boil, and boil for 1 minute. Immediately remove the saucepan from the heat and let the eggs sit in the hot water for an additional 12 minutes. Drain the eggs and rinse them under cold water to stop the cooking process. Store in the refrigerator.

PER SERVING
Macronutrients: Fat 69%; Protein 18%; Carbs 13%
Calories: 563; Total Fat: 43g; Protein: 25g; Total Carbs: 19g; Fiber: 10g; Net Carbs: 9g

CHOPPED SALAD

YIELD: *1 serving*

4 cherry tomatoes, halved

¼ medium red onion, cut into half-inch pieces

¼ green bell pepper, cut into half-inch pieces

¼ cucumber, peeled and cut into half-inch pieces

4 kalamata olives, pitted and halved

2 tablespoons Italian Vinaigrette, divided (page 90)

1 cooked boneless chicken thigh, cut into half-inch pieces

1 tablespoon feta cheese (optional)

½ avocado, cut into half-inch pieces (optional)

Chopped salads are great because they harmoniously combine the flavors and textures of a variety of ingredients. Using crisp vegetables and diced chicken as the base and drizzling it with homemade Italian Vinaigrette will make this your new favorite salad.

1. Combine the tomatoes, onion, bell pepper, cucumber, olives, and 1 tablespoon of Italian Vinaigrette in a bowl and stir gently, making sure the dressing is distributed evenly.

2. Add the chicken, and drizzle the remaining 1 tablespoon of dressing over the salad.

3. Season with salt and freshly ground black pepper to taste.

4. Add the feta cheese and avocado (if using).

CKL TIP: If you're serving this salad to a group of people, it looks beautiful to keep the elements segmented in lines or quadrants. If you decide to do this, place each element in the bowl first and add the dressing on top, then mix the salad together just before serving (but after presenting it to the group)!

PER SERVING
Macronutrients: Fat 65%; Protein 19%; Carbs 16%
Calories: 371; Total Fat: 27g; Protein: 17g; Total Carbs: 15g; Fiber: 3g; Net Carbs: 12g

ZESTY CHICKEN TENDER SALAD

YIELD: *1 serving*

Juice of 1 lime

1 teaspoon Dijon mustard

1 teaspoon Italian
Seasoning (page 82)

1 garlic clove, minced

½ teaspoon pink
Himalayan salt

1 tablespoon extra-virgin
olive oil

2 cups fresh spinach

3 cooked chicken
tenderloins

The dressing is the star of this simple salad with a spinach base. Add some chopped cucumbers, onions, celery, or broccoli to give it a little extra crunch.

1. Put the lime juice, mustard, Italian Seasoning, garlic, salt, and oil into a blender; process until smooth.

2. Place the spinach on a plate or in a bowl. Arrange the chicken tenders on top of the spinach, and drizzle with the blended dressing.

PER SERVING

Macronutrients: Fat 51%; Protein 39%; Carbs 10%
Calories: 284; Total Fat: 16g; Protein: 28g; Total Carbs: 7g; Fiber: 2g; Net Carbs: 5g

SPINACH BACON SALAD

YIELD: *1 serving*

1 garlic clove, minced

¼ teaspoon pink Himalayan salt

1 tablespoon apple cider vinegar

1 teaspoon Dijon mustard

1 tablespoon extra-virgin olive oil

2 cups fresh spinach

1 hard-boiled egg, peeled and quartered

2 bacon slices, cooked and crumbled

Bacon on salad is a game changer. It adds a satisfying, salty crunch that can't be beat. Combined with spinach, eggs, and a tasty dressing, you have the perfect keto meal.

1. With the flat side of a chef's knife, mash the minced garlic, cover it with the salt, and combine to form a paste. Place the mixture in a medium bowl.

2. Whisk in the vinegar and mustard.

3. Gradually add the oil, whisking until well combined.

4. Season with freshly ground black pepper.

5. Put the spinach, egg, and bacon in a large salad bowl. Cover with the dressing, and toss to combine.

CKL TIP: If you can find it, buy bacon that is sugar-free, uncured, and with few or no nitrates or preservatives.

PER SERVING
Macronutrients: Fat 74%; Protein 21%; Carbs 5%
Calories: 423; Total Fat: 35g; Protein: 22g; Total Carbs: 5g; Fiber: 2g; Net Carbs: 3g

GRANDMA'S BROCCOLI SALAD

YIELD: *1 serving*

1 tablespoon no-sugar-added mayonnaise

1 tablespoon apple cider vinegar

½ teaspoon stevia *or* 4 drops liquid stevia extract (optional)

1½ cups broccoli florets

2 bacon slices, cooked and crumbled

¼ medium red onion, diced

¼ cup raw sliced almonds

When I was young, the only time I would willingly eat broccoli was when my grandma made her broccoli salad. This keto version substitutes pure stevia for the white sugar, which provides the perfect amount of sweetness to offset the tanginess of the mayo and vinegar.

1. In a small bowl, mix the mayonnaise, vinegar, and stevia (if using) until well combined.

2. Season the dressing with salt and freshly ground black pepper to taste.

3. In a large bowl, combine the broccoli, bacon, onion, and almonds.

4. Pour the dressing over the broccoli mixture and stir until evenly coated.

5. Cover and refrigerate for at least 1 hour before serving.

PER SERVING
Macronutrients: Fat 69%; Protein 18%; Carbs 13%
Calories: 511; Total Fat: 39g; Protein: 23g; Total Carbs: 17g; Fiber: 8g; Net Carbs: 9g

STEAK SALAD

YIELD: *1 serving*

1 (6-ounce) skirt steak

¼ cup coconut aminos

2 tablespoons avocado oil

2 cups mixed greens

4 cherry tomatoes, halved

2 radishes, sliced

2 tablespoons extra-virgin olive oil

Juice of ½ lemon

Steak is one of the most flavorful meats that you can cook, so it makes a wonderful salad topper. Dress the salad with just a little lemon juice and extra-virgin olive oil to allow the savory flavors of the marinated steak to shine.

1. Marinate the steak in the coconut aminos for 5 minutes.
2. In a skillet, heat the avocado oil over high heat.
3. Cook the marinated steak to your desired level of doneness.
4. Place the steak on a plate, and let it sit for 5 minutes.
5. Prepare the salad by tossing the mixed greens, tomatoes, and radishes in a bowl with the olive oil and lemon juice.
6. Season with salt and freshly ground black pepper to taste.
7. Cut the steak into slices, and arrange them on top of the salad.

PER SERVING
Macronutrients: Fat 77%; Protein 17%; Carbs 6%
Calories: 792; Total Fat: 68g; Protein: 33g; Total Carbs: 12g; Fiber: 4g; Net Carbs: 8g

CHICKEN TORTILLA SOUP

YIELD: *2 servings (2 cups per serving)*

2 tablespoons avocado oil

¼ medium white
onion, diced

¼ red bell pepper, diced

1 garlic clove, minced

½ cup diced tomatoes,
fresh or canned

1 tablespoon Taco
Seasoning (page 84)

4 cups chicken broth

1 tablespoon minced
fresh cilantro

3 cooked boneless chicken
thighs, shredded
with a fork

Juice of ½ lime

½ avocado, pitted, peeled,
and diced

I can't get enough of this soup! I always make a triple batch
so I can eat it all week long. My favorite topping is freshly
diced avocado or a dollop of sour cream.

1. In a medium pot, heat the oil over medium heat.

2. Add the onion, bell pepper, and garlic, and sauté 5 to
    7 minutes until soft.

3. Add the tomatoes and Taco Seasoning; stir well.

4. Let cook for 2 to 3 minutes.

5. Add the chicken broth and cilantro, and stir everything
    together.

6. Bring the soup up to a boil, then reduce the heat to low
    and let it simmer for 20 minutes.

7. Add the cooked chicken and lime juice to the pot, and stir
    together until everything is combined.

8. Garnish with the diced avocado, more lime juice, or extra
    cilantro.

PER SERVING

Macronutrients: Fat 70%; Protein 23%; Carbs 7%
Calories: 529; Total Fat: 41g; Protein: 31g; Total Carbs: 9g; Fiber: 4g; Net Carbs: 5g

PREP TIME: 10 minutes
COOK TIME: 2 hours,
10 minutes

SLOW COOKER KETO CHILI

YIELD: *2 servings (2 cups per serving)*

1 tablespoon avocado oil

¼ medium white onion, diced

¼ green bell pepper, diced

2 garlic cloves, minced

12 ounces ground beef

1 (12-ounce) can tomato sauce

1 tablespoon coconut aminos

2 cups beef broth

½ teaspoon ground cumin

½ teaspoon garlic powder

¼ teaspoon chili powder

¼ teaspoon paprika

¼ teaspoon dried oregano

¼ teaspoon cayenne pepper

¼ teaspoon freshly ground black pepper

¼ teaspoon pink Himalayan salt

If you are looking for a worthy crowd-pleaser on game day, you've come to the right place. Be sure to adjust the recipe based on how many people you are feeding. This comes together in a slow cooker, so you can make it in advance and keep it warm until you're ready to serve it. I love creating a toppings bar with cheddar cheese, pickled jalapeños, diced onion, and sour cream and letting people create their own personalized chili bowl.

1. In a large skillet, heat the oil over medium heat.
2. Add the onion, bell pepper, and garlic, and sauté for 5 to 7 minutes, until soft.
3. Add the ground beef and cook until it is browned and no longer pink.
4. Transfer the mixture to a slow cooker.
5. Add the tomato sauce, coconut aminos, broth, cumin, garlic powder, chili powder, paprika, oregano, cayenne, black pepper, and salt.
6. Stir to combine everything.
7. Cook on high for 2 hours, stirring occasionally.

PER SERVING
Macronutrients: Fat 69%; Protein 21%; Carbs 10%
Calories: 663; Total Fat: 51g; Protein: 35g; Total Carbs: 16g; Fiber: 4g; Net Carbs: 12g

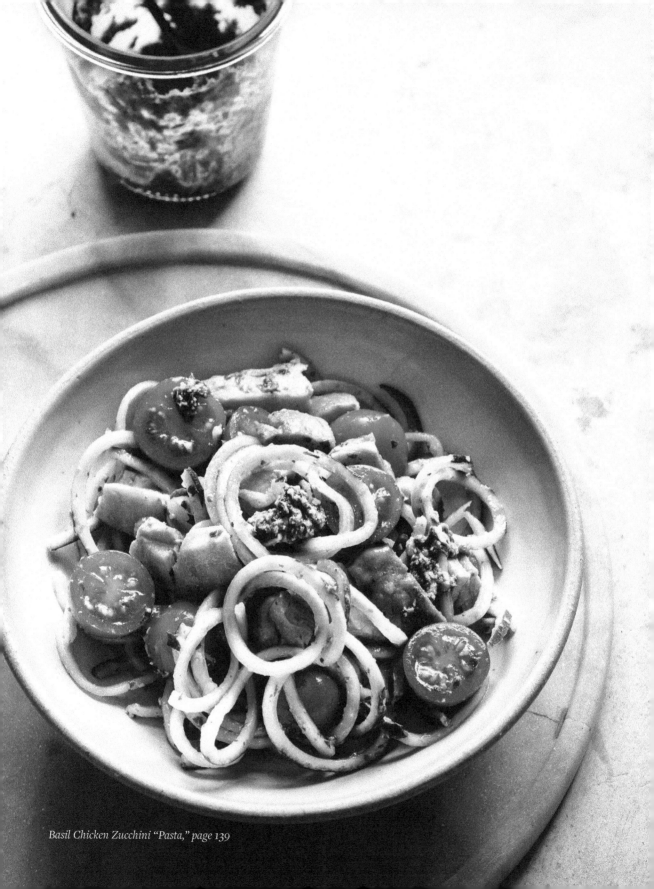

Basil Chicken Zucchini "Pasta," page 139

10

SEAFOOD & POULTRY

ROASTED SHRIMP & VEGGIES

YIELD: *1 serving*

½ zucchini, cut into
half-moons

¼ red onion, cut into
half-inch pieces

¼ red bell pepper, cut into
half-inch pieces

2 garlic cloves,
minced, divided

¼ teaspoon
paprika, divided

2 tablespoons grass-fed
butter or ghee,
melted, divided

6 ounces peeled shrimp

½ lemon, cut into wedges,
for garnish

You'll only get two dishes dirty while cooking this veggie-packed dinner. The paprika adds a delicious spice to the shrimp and veggies. Plus, you can't go wrong with garlic, lemon, and butter when it comes to seafood. So good.

1. Preheat the oven to 425°F; line a baking sheet with parchment paper.

2. Place the zucchini, onion, and bell pepper in a large bowl, and sprinkle with half the garlic and half the paprika. Add 1 tablespoon of the butter.

3. Spread the vegetables onto the prepared baking sheet, and bake for 12 to 15 minutes.

4. Put the shrimp in the same bowl that was used for the vegetables, and mix in the remaining garlic, paprika, and butter.

5. Combine to completely coat the shrimp.

6. Add the shrimp to the baking sheet with the vegetables, and bake for 5 additional minutes, until the shrimp are pink.

7. Spoon the shrimp and vegetables into a bowl; garnish with the lemon wedges.

PER SERVING

Macronutrients: Fat 53%; Protein 37%; Carbs 10%
Calories: 421; Total Fat: 25g; Protein: 39g; Total Carbs: 10g; Fiber: 3g; Net Carbs: 7g

LEMON SALMON & ASPARAGUS

YIELD: *1 serving*

2 tablespoons avocado
oil, divided

2 garlic cloves, minced

1 (6-ounce) salmon fillet

Juice of ½ lemon

6 asparagus spears, woody
ends removed

Half a lemon, sliced thinly

One of the first meals I prepared when starting the keto diet was this one, and I was blown away by how simple and satisfying it was. Making it gave me the confidence I needed to know eating like this is a true lifestyle.

1. Preheat the oven to 425°F; line a baking sheet with parchment paper.

2. Combine 1 tablespoon of avocado oil and the garlic in a bowl.

3. Place the salmon on the prepared baking sheet.

4. Rub the salmon with the garlic and oil mixture until it is evenly coated.

5. Squeeze the lemon juice over the salmon, and season with salt and freshly ground black pepper.

6. Arrange the asparagus around the salmon in a single layer, drizzle the spears with the remaining 1 tablespoon of avocado oil, and place the lemon slices over them.

7. Roast for 12 to 15 minutes, until the salmon is cooked through to your liking.

PER SERVING
Macronutrients: Fat 67%; Protein 27%; Carbs 6%
Calories: 527; Total Fat: 39g; Protein: 36g; Total Carbs: 8g; Fiber: 3g; Net Carbs: 5g

ASIAN-STYLE SALMON

YIELD: *1 serving*

1 teaspoon Dijon mustard

1 teaspoon coconut aminos

1 teaspoon avocado oil

1 garlic clove, minced

¼ teaspoon freshly grated ginger root

1 (6-ounce) salmon fillet

If you haven't cooked with fresh ginger, you are definitely missing out. The flavor adds zing to any dish and pairs particularly well with salmon. Peel the ginger before grating it with a small grater or microplane.

1. Whisk together the mustard, coconut aminos, oil, garlic, and ginger in a small bowl.

2. Drizzle the marinade over the salmon, and allow it to sit for 10 minutes.

3. Heat a skillet over medium-high heat.

4. Place the salmon in the skillet; discard any leftover marinade.

5. Cook for 4 to 5 minutes, depending on the thickness of the fish.

6. Turn the salmon carefully with a spatula, then cook for another 4 to 5 minutes or until it is cooked through to your liking.

PER SERVING
Macronutrients: Fat 60%; Protein 37%; Carbs 3%
Calories: 355; Total Fat: 23g; Protein: 34g; Total Carbs: 3g; Fiber: 0g; Net Carbs: 3g

PAN-FRIED SCALLOPS

YIELD: 1 serving

½ tablespoon avocado oil

1 tablespoon grass-fed butter or ghee

6 ounces scallops, rinsed with cold water and patted dry

Scallops are my go-to protein when I don't have much time to cook. They brown in just a few minutes and I can put them on top of a crisp salad or serve them with a simple keto side dish. The only seasoning I give them is a little salt and pepper to preserve their natural flavor.

1. In a large skillet, heat the oil and butter over high heat until it begins to smoke.

2. Generously season the scallops with salt and freshly ground black pepper.

3. Gently add the scallops to the pan, making sure they are not touching.

4. Sear the scallops for 90 seconds on each side.

5. The scallops should have a nice golden crust on each side and be translucent in the center.

PER SERVING
Macronutrients: Fat 60%; Protein 38%; Carbs 2%
Calories: 304; Total Fat: 20g; Protein: 29g; Total Carbs: 4g; Fiber: 0g; Net Carbs: 4g

LETTUCE-WRAPPED CHICKEN BURGER

YIELD: *1 serving*

1 tablespoon avocado oil

6 ounces ground chicken

1 avocado, pitted, peeled, and sliced

4 Bibb lettuce leaves

Obviously, standard burger buns are not an option in the keto world, but don't fear! You can still enjoy that handheld burger with the help of a few crisp Bibb lettuce leaves. Dress your burger as you like with mustard, mayo, tomato slices, sprouts, or no-sugar-added pickles. Wrap the whole thing in the lettuce leaves, and enjoy.

1. In a large skillet, heat the oil over medium heat.

2. Form the ground chicken into a patty and season with salt and freshly ground black pepper.

3. Add the chicken patty to the skillet and cook until it is nicely browned on each side and no longer pink in the center, 3 to 5 minutes on each side.

4. Top the patty with the sliced avocado, and wrap it in the lettuce leaves.

PER SERVING

Macronutrients: Fat 71%; Protein 19%; Carbs 10%
Calories: 682; Total Fat: 54g; Protein: 33g; Total Carbs: 16g; Fiber: 12g; Net Carbs: 4g

CHICKEN STRIP WRAPS

YIELD: *1 serving*

1 egg

1 teaspoon Italian
Seasoning (page 82)

1 tablespoon avocado oil

2 boneless chicken thighs,
cut into thin strips

2 Bibb lettuce leaves

I've found that in addition to replacing the burger buns, Bibb lettuce makes for great wraps, as well. Dipping the chicken in the egg gives it a delicate coating. I like to serve these wraps with a dollop of Keto Ranch (page 91).

1. In a medium bowl, whisk the egg. Add the Italian Seasoning and whisk thoroughly. Season with a little salt and freshly ground black pepper.

2. In a large skillet, heat the oil over medium heat.

3. Coat the chicken strips in the egg mixture.

4. Add the chicken to the skillet and cook for 5 minutes, turning occasionally, until fully cooked.

5. Wrap the chicken in the lettuce leaves.

PER SERVING
Macronutrients: Fat 73%; Protein 26%; Carbs 1%
Calories: 544; Total Fat: 44g; Protein: 36g; Total Carbs: 1g; Fiber: 0g; Net Carbs: 1g

TURKEY TACO BOWL

YIELD: 1 serving

1 tablespoon avocado oil

¼ medium red onion, diced

6 ounces ground turkey

1 tablespoon Taco
 Seasoning (page 84)

2 cups mixed greens

1 serving Guacamole
 (page 92)

I love Taco bowls! It's such fun to mix and match the ingredients. The combination here is probably my favorite, but sometimes I swap out the ground turkey for beef or chicken. I've also been known to substitute the mixed greens for Mexican Cauliflower Rice (page 111). Be as creative as you like, and discover your favorite combination.

1. In a large skillet, heat the oil over medium-high heat.

2. Add the onion and sauté for 5 to 7 minutes, until soft.

3. Add the ground turkey and cook until it's no longer pink, breaking the meat into small pieces as it cooks, about 5 minutes.

4. Add the Taco Seasoning, and stir the mixture constantly for 1 minute. It will be crumbly (that's okay).

5. Place the mixed greens in a bowl, and top with the turkey mixture. Dollop with the Guacamole.

CKL TIP: If you would like additional toppings, try adding diced tomatoes, lime wedges, black olives, or a dollop of full-fat sour cream to your bowl.

PER SERVING
Macronutrients: Fat 64%; Protein 23%; Carbs 13%
Calories: 581; Total Fat: 41g; Protein: 34g; Total Carbs: 19g; Fiber: 10g; Net Carbs: 9g

BASIL CHICKEN ZUCCHINI "PASTA"

YIELD: *1 serving*

1 tablespoon grass-fed butter or ghee

2 boneless chicken thighs, cubed

¼ medium white onion, diced

2 garlic cloves, minced

½ zucchini, peeled into thin ribbons or spiralized

1 teaspoon avocado oil

¼ cup Basil Pesto (page 87)

4 cherry tomatoes, halved

This "pasta" is actually thinly sliced zucchini that tastes great served warm or cold, which makes it extremely versatile. Be careful not to overcook the zucchini noodles, though—aim for an al dente texture. If you tolerate dairy well, top it with some fresh mozzarella.

1. In a skillet, melt the butter over medium-high heat.
2. Add the chicken and onion, and cook for several minutes, until the chicken begins to brown.
3. Add the garlic and cook for another 2 to 3 minutes, until the chicken is cooked through.
4. Turn the heat down to low.
5. In a medium bowl, coat the zucchini in the oil.
6. Add the zucchini to the skillet and cook for 1 minute, stirring occasionally.
7. Transfer the mixture to a medium bowl, and toss with the Basil Pesto and tomatoes.

CKL TIP: If you don't have a spiralizer, look for prepackaged zucchini noodles in the produce section of the grocery store. Or, using a veggie peeler, peel the zucchini lengthwise into thin strips resembling noodles. You can buy a spiralizer online for $20 to $30.

PER SERVING
Macronutrients: Fat 76%; Protein 17%; Carbs 7%
Calories: 875; Total Fat: 74g; Protein: 37g; Total Carbs: 15g; Fiber: 8g; Net Carbs: 7g

BALSAMIC CHICKEN

YIELD: 1 serving

1 teaspoon balsamic
vinegar

2 tablespoons avocado
oil, divided

1 teaspoon Dijon mustard

1 garlic clove, minced

Pinch red pepper flakes

2 boneless chicken thighs

4 asparagus spears,
woody ends removed

4 cherry tomatoes, halved

I have always loved balsamic vinegar, so it made sense to me to create a dish that showcases its sweet and tart flavor. Be sure to buy a balsamic brand that has no added sugars. Anything else is not keto.

1. In a small bowl, combine the vinegar, 1 tablespoon of oil, the mustard, garlic, and red pepper flakes. Whisk until fully combined, and set aside.

2. In a large skillet over medium heat, add the remaining 1 tablespoon of oil.

3. Thoroughly season the chicken thighs with salt and freshly ground black pepper, and add them to the skillet, searing each side for 3 minutes or until golden.

4. Remove the chicken from the skillet, and set it on a plate.

5. Next, add the asparagus and tomatoes to the same skillet, season with more salt and pepper to taste, and cook for about 5 minutes, until the asparagus is bright green and the tomatoes are slightly wilted.

6. Move the vegetables to one side of the skillet, and return the chicken to the skillet.

7. Pour the balsamic mixture over the chicken and vegetables.

8. Toss everything together, and cook for about 5 minutes more, until the chicken is fully cooked through and the vinaigrette has thickened.

PER SERVING
Macronutrients: Fat 75%; Protein 20%; Carbs 5%
Calories: 650; Total Fat: 54g; Protein: 33g; Total Carbs: 8g; Fiber: 5g; Net Carbs: 3g

TURKEY MEATBALLS

YIELD: *1 serving*

1 egg

6 ounces ground turkey

¼ cup almond flour

1 tablespoon Italian Seasoning (page 82)

½ cup Italian Marinara Sauce (page 86)

Almond flour is a great substitute for breadcrumbs in this meatball recipe. I usually make my Italian Marinara Sauce (page 86) while the meatballs are baking to perfection in the oven. Serve with zucchini noodles, spaghetti squash, garlicky kale, or a simple salad.

1. Preheat the oven to 425°F; line a baking sheet with parchment paper.
2. In a small bowl, beat the egg.
3. Add the ground turkey, almond flour, and Italian Seasoning to the egg.
4. Mix together with your (clean!) hands until fully combined.
5. Form into three meatballs, and place them on the prepared baking sheet.
6. Bake for 30 minutes.
7. Place the meatballs in a bowl, and top with the Italian Marinara Sauce.

PER SERVING
Macronutrients: Fat 52%; Protein 41%; Carbs 7%
Calories: 382; Total Fat: 22g; Protein: 39g; Total Carbs: 7g; Fiber: 3g; Net Carbs: 4g

PREP TIME: 5 minutes
COOK TIME: 25 minutes

BACON-WRAPPED CHICKEN

YIELD: *1 serving*

2 garlic cloves, minced

1 tablespoon avocado oil

2 boneless chicken thighs

4 uncooked bacon slices

Bacon makes everything taste better, and this dish is a perfect example. The crispness of the bacon combined with the juiciness of the chicken makes for a powerful combo that will soon be a family favorite.

1. Preheat the oven to 400°F; line a baking sheet with parchment paper.
2. Mix the garlic and oil together in a bowl.
3. Coat the chicken thighs in the garlic mixture, and wrap each thigh in 2 slices of bacon.
4. Place the chicken on the prepared baking sheet, and bake for about 25 minutes, flipping the pieces halfway through, until the bacon is crisp.

PER SERVING
Macronutrients: Fat 72%; Protein 27%; Carbs 1%
Calories: 887; Total Fat: 71g; Protein: 59g; Total Carbs: 3g; Fiber: 0g; Net Carbs: 3g

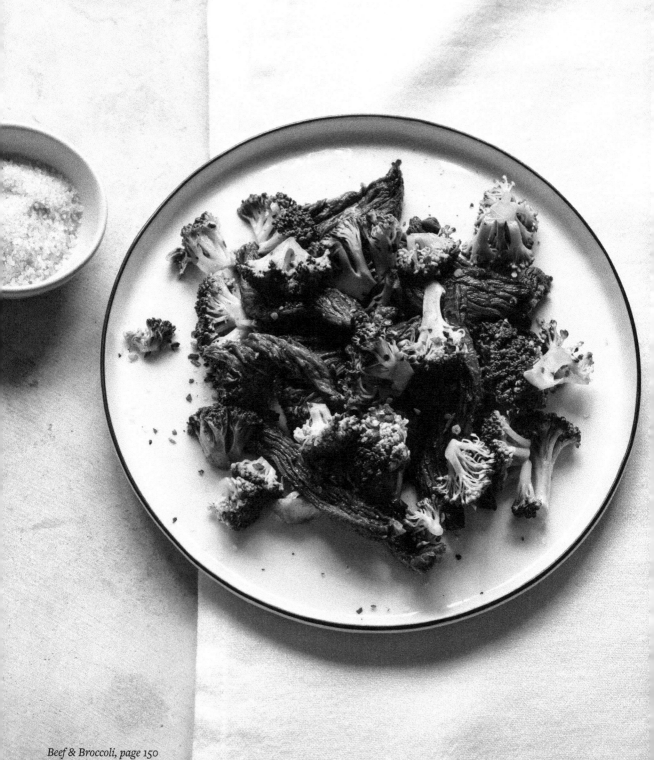

Beef & Broccoli, page 150

Chapter

11

BEEF & PORK

STEAK FAJITAS

YIELD: *1 serving*

1 tablespoon avocado oil

¼ medium white onion, thinly sliced

¼ green bell pepper, thinly sliced

6 ounces skirt steak, cut into thin, 2-inch strips

1 tablespoon Taco Seasoning (page 84)

½ cup Guacamole (page 92)

Is there anything better than a sizzling skillet of fajitas? I love using a gorgeous piece of skirt steak as the centerpiece of this dish. It cooks fast and absorbs all the spices beautifully. These fajitas taste great alongside a serving of Mexican Cauliflower Rice (page 111).

1. In a large skillet, heat the oil over medium-high heat.
2. Add the onion and bell pepper, and sauté until the vegetables begin to soften.
3. Add the steak and Taco Seasoning, and cook until the vegetables are tender and the steak is cooked to your desired doneness.
4. Top the steak and vegetables with the Guacamole.

CKL TIP: For more toppings, try diced tomatoes, lime wedges, or a dollop of full-fat sour cream.

PER SERVING
Macronutrients: Fat 65%; Protein 24%; Carbs 11%
Calories: 543; Total Fat: 39g; Protein: 33g; Total Carbs: 15g; Fiber: 8g; Net Carbs: 7g

MINI BURGER SLIDERS

YIELD: *1 serving*

6 ounces ground beef

1 zucchini, cut into
  8 half-inch-thick slices

1 cheddar cheese slice, cut
  into 4 squares (optional)

1 avocado

Mini burger sliders may look small, but they pack a powerful flavor punch. I like to make a big batch of these when I host a family gathering. I'll put out a bunch of different toppings and let everyone pick their favorites.

1. Preheat the oven to 400°F; line a baking sheet with parchment paper.

2. In a medium bowl, season the ground beef with salt and freshly ground black pepper, and mix thoroughly.

3. Form four small, slider-size patties, and place them on the prepared baking sheet. Arrange the zucchini slices around the patties on the baking sheet.

4. Bake the patties and zucchini slices for about 5 minutes, flip them, and then continue to bake for another 5 minutes.

5. Place one square of cheddar cheese (if using), on top of each patty during the last minute of baking. Watch carefully so the cheese does not burn.

6. Remove the sliders from the oven, and place them on a plate.

7. Slice or mash the avocado, and place some on top of each patty.

8. Assemble the sliders, using the zucchini slices as buns.

CKL TIP: You can also use the grill for this recipe. For toppings, add sliced tomato, diced onion, dill pickles, and mustard.

PER SERVING
Macronutrients: Fat 74%; Protein 17%; Carbs 9%
Calories: 950; Total Fat: 78g; Protein: 40g; Total Carbs: 22g; Fiber: 14g;
  Net Carbs: 8g

PORK TENDERLOIN

YIELD: *1 serving*

2 tablespoons coconut oil

6 ounces pork tenderloin

Two words: simple perfection. Despite its simplicity, I don't think there is a better way to eat pork tenderloin— the coconut oil gives it a subtle, sweet flavor I just can't get enough of. Serve this with any of my keto side dishes for a complete meal.

1. In a large skillet, melt the coconut oil over medium-high heat.
2. Rub the pork with salt and freshly ground black pepper.
3. Place the pork tenderloin in the skillet and cook for 4 to 5 minutes on each side, depending on the thickness.
4. Make a small cut into the middle of the tenderloin to make sure it is fully cooked on the inside.

CKL TIP: If you have any leftover fresh herbs, chop them up and use them as an edible garnish to make this extra delicious.

PER SERVING
Macronutrients: Fat 66%; Protein 34%; Carbs 0%
Calories: 423; Total Fat: 31g; Protein: 36g; Total Carbs: 0g; Fiber: 0g; Net Carbs: 0g

ITALIAN ZOODLES

YIELD: *1 serving*

6 ounces ground beef

1 tablespoon avocado oil

2 garlic cloves, minced

¼ medium white
onion, diced

½ cup Italian Marinara
Sauce (page 86)

1 cup fresh spinach

½ zucchini, peeled
into thin ribbons or
spiralized

My husband's all-time favorite meal is spaghetti Bolognese, so I created a keto version of this Italian classic (with a few veggies added in, of course). The heat of the sauce will cook the zucchini noodles, so there is no need to cook them ahead of time.

1. In a medium bowl, season the ground beef with salt and freshly ground black pepper, and mix thoroughly.
2. In a large skillet, heat the oil over medium-high heat.
3. Add the garlic, and let it sizzle for 20 to 30 seconds.
4. Add the onion and sauté for 3 minutes.
5. Add the ground beef, and cook until it's no longer pink, about 5 minutes.
6. Add the Italian Marinara Sauce and the spinach, stirring to combine.
7. Reduce the heat to low, and simmer for 15 minutes.
8. Serve over the zucchini.

CKL TIP: If you don't have a spiralizer, you can just slice your zucchini into thin half moons and prepare the recipe the same way.

PER SERVING
Macronutrients: Fat 73%; Protein 18%; Carbs 9%
Calories: 701; Total Fat: 57g; Protein: 31g; Total Carbs: 16g; Fiber: 4g; Net Carbs: 12g

---

BEEF & BROCCOLI

YIELD: *1 serving*

1 tablespoon coconut oil

6 ounces skirt steak, cut into thin, 2-inch strips

2 garlic cloves, minced

½ teaspoon peeled and minced ginger root

1½ cups broccoli florets

¼ cup water

¼ cup coconut aminos

½ teaspoon apple cider vinegar

Juice of ½ lemon

Pinch red pepper flakes (optional)

Skip the Chinese takeout and make an upgraded keto version of this popular dish. My clients rave about this recipe, and it will most likely become a keto staple for you. Serve it on its own or with cauliflower rice for an indulgent, yet guilt-free, meal.

1. In a large skillet, melt the coconut oil over medium-high heat.
2. Sauté the steak for 5 to 7 minutes.
3. Remove the steak, and set it aside on a plate.
4. Lower the heat to medium, and add the garlic and ginger; cook and stir until fragrant, about 1 minute.
5. Add the broccoli and cook for 2 minutes, until lightly browned.
6. Add the water, cover, and reduce the heat to medium-low.
7. Cook for 10 minutes, stirring occasionally, until the broccoli is tender.
8. Add the coconut aminos, vinegar, lemon juice, red pepper flakes (if using), and the reserved steak to the broccoli.
9. Sauté, tossing to combine, for 1 to 2 minutes.
10. Season with salt and freshly ground black pepper to taste.

PER SERVING
Macronutrients: Fat 51%; Protein 31%; Carbs 18%
Calories: 458; Total Fat: 26g; Protein: 35g; Total Carbs: 21g; Fiber: 4g; Net Carbs: 17g

EGG ROLL IN A BOWL

YIELD: *1 serving*

6 ounces ground pork

2 cups cabbage coleslaw mix or shredded cabbage

1 garlic clove, minced

1 teaspoon peeled and minced ginger root

1 teaspoon coconut aminos

1 scallion, finely sliced

1 teaspoon sesame oil

Who says you have to give up egg rolls when you go keto? The best part of the egg roll is the filling anyway, so this recipe focuses on the good stuff.

1. Heat a large skillet over medium heat.

2. Add the ground pork and cook, stirring often to crumble it, until it is cooked through.

3. Add the cabbage, garlic, ginger, and coconut aminos, and cook for 3 to 4 minutes or until the cabbage softens.

4. Transfer to a plate, sprinkle with the scallion, and drizzle with the sesame oil.

PER SERVING
Macronutrients: Fat 69%; Protein 22%; Carbs 9%
Calories: 463; Total Fat: 35g; Protein: 26g; Total Carbs: 11g; Fiber: 5g; Net Carbs: 6g

RIB EYE STEAK

YIELD: *1 serving*

1 (6-ounce) rib eye steak, about 1 inch thick

2 tablespoons avocado oil, divided

1 tablespoon Garlic & Herb Compound Butter (page 85)

Looking for a showstopper entrée? Look no further than a classic rib eye steak. If you use this technique for cooking steak, it will come out perfectly every time. Don't forget to top the steak with the savory Garlic & Herb Compound Butter to make the flavor out of this world.

1. Pat both sides of the steak dry with a paper towel.
2. Drizzle the steak with 1 tablespoon of the oil, and season with salt and freshly ground black pepper.
3. Preheat the oven to broil.
4. In an ovenproof skillet or a cast iron pan, heat the remaining 1 tablespoon of oil over medium-high heat.
5. Place the steak in the middle of the skillet, and cook on one side until a dark crust has formed, about 1 minute.
6. Using tongs, flip the steak and cook for an additional minute.
7. Transfer the skillet to the oven, and cook until the steak is cooked to your desired doneness, 4 to 5 minutes for medium-rare, flipping once after 3 minutes.
8. Be careful! Use pot holders when removing the skillet from the oven.
9. Transfer the steak to a plate, and let it rest for 3 to 5 minutes.
10. Top with the butter.

PER SERVING
Macronutrients: Fat 79%; Protein 21%; Carbs 0%
Calories: 579; Total Fat: 51g; Protein: 30g; Total Carbs: 0g; Fiber: 0g; Net Carbs: 0g

CHEESEBURGER MEAT LOAF

YIELD: 1 serving

6 ounces ground beef

1 egg, beaten

¼ medium white
onion, diced

1 teaspoon pink
Himalayan salt

1 teaspoon garlic powder

¼ cup cubed
cheddar cheese

2 tablespoons
tomato paste

1 tablespoon
yellow mustard

1 tablespoon
coconut aminos

Who needs a bun when you can take all the goodness of a classic juicy cheeseburger and transform it into a delicious meat loaf? Double the recipe, and you'll have plenty of leftovers for the next day. You are going to want them!

1. Preheat the oven to 350°F; line a baking sheet with parchment paper.

2. In a large bowl, combine the ground beef, egg, onion, salt, garlic, and cheese.

3. Using your hands, gently mix the ingredients, being careful not to overmix, which can make the meat loaf tough.

4. Place the mixture on the prepared baking sheet, and form it into a meat loaf shape.

5. Transfer the meat loaf to the oven, and bake for 30 minutes.

6. In a small bowl, whisk together the tomato paste, mustard, and coconut aminos until fully combined.

7. Remove the meat loaf from the oven, and spread the sauce mixture over the top evenly with a spoon.

8. Place the meat loaf back in the oven, and bake for another 15 minutes or until cooked through and browned on top.

PER SERVING
Macronutrients: Fat 70%; Protein 23%; Carbs 7%
Calories: 737; Total Fat: 57g; Protein: 42g; Total Carbs: 14g; Fiber: 4g; Net Carbs: 10g

PORK FRIED RICE

YIELD: *1 serving*

½ head cauliflower, cut into small florets

1 tablespoon avocado oil

1 (6-ounce) pork tenderloin, cut into thin strips

1 tablespoon grass-fed butter or ghee

1 scallion, finely sliced (green and white parts divided)

1 teaspoon peeled and minced ginger root

1 garlic clove, minced

1 egg, beaten

1 tablespoon coconut aminos

1 teaspoon sesame oil

My non-keto friends are always shocked when I make this for them and they realize the "rice" is actually cauliflower. This dish is a fan favorite that will not disappoint—whether you are eating keto or not.

1. Place the cauliflower florets in a food processor, and process until the mixture resembles rice.

2. In a large skillet, heat the oil over medium heat.

3. Sauté the pork strips for 4 to 5 minutes, then transfer them to a plate and set aside.

4. In the same skillet, combine the butter, cauliflower "rice," and the white parts of the scallion, and cook for about 5 minutes or until the cauliflower begins to soften slightly.

5. Add the ginger and garlic, and stir for about 30 seconds.

6. Add the beaten egg and cook, stirring continuously.

7. Add the pork and coconut aminos, and cook for another 2 minutes, stirring continuously.

8. Remove from the heat, and stir in the sesame oil and green parts of the scallion.

PER SERVING
Macronutrients: Fat 65%; Protein 28%; Carbs 7%
Calories: 565; Total Fat: 41g; Protein: 39g; Total Carbs: 10g; Fiber: 4g; Net Carbs: 6g

MARINATED FLANK STEAK

YIELD: *1 serving*

1 tablespoon avocado oil

1 garlic clove, minced

1 tablespoon red
wine vinegar

1 tablespoon
coconut aminos

½ teaspoon pink
Himalayan salt

6 ounces flank steak

Nothing is better than a tender, marinated steak. The steak needs to marinate overnight, but it is well worth waiting for. Coconut aminos, which fills in for soy sauce, is the perfect partner for the steak.

1. In a large zip-top bag or sealed container, mix together the oil, garlic, vinegar, coconut aminos, and salt.

2. Add the flank steak, and close the bag. Massage the bag to make sure both sides of the steak are coated generously with the marinade.

3. Refrigerate overnight.

4. When you are ready to cook, remove the steak from the refrigerator and let it sit at room temperature for 20 minutes.

5. Preheat a large skillet over medium-high heat.

6. Cook the steak for 3 to 4 minutes on each side for medium-rare.

7. Transfer the steak to a cutting board, and let it rest for 10 minutes before serving.

PER SERVING
Macronutrients: Fat 58%; Protein 39%; Carbs 3%
Calories: 393; Total Fat: 25g; Protein: 38g; Total Carbs: 4g; Fiber: 1g; Net Carbs: 3g

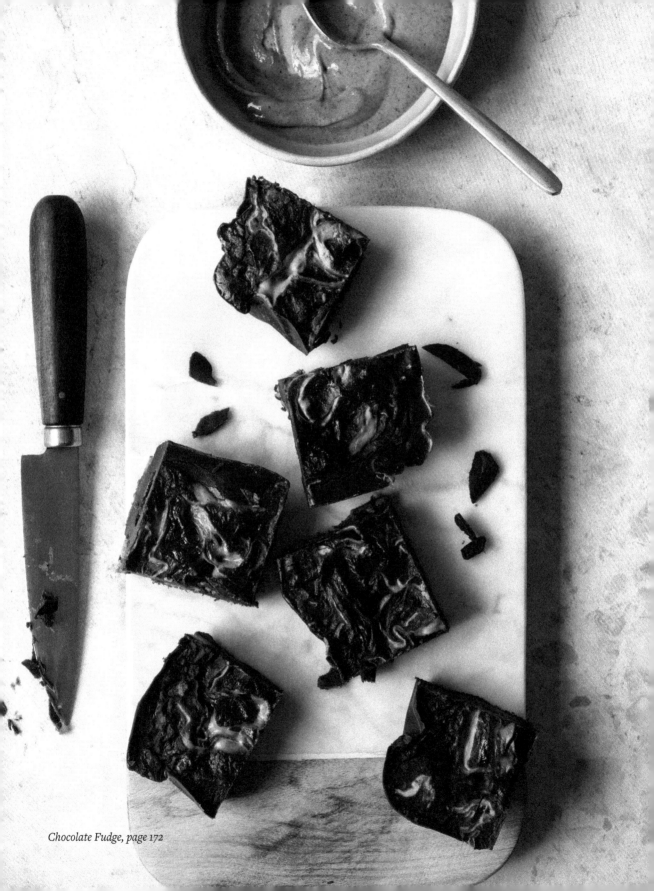

Chocolate Fudge, page 172

BEVERAGES & DESSERTS

CREAMY COFFEE

YIELD: 1 serving (16.5 ounces)

1 cup brewed black coffee

1 cup unsweetened full-fat coconut milk

½ tablespoon grass-fed butter or ghee

½ tablespoon MCT oil

Swap out that sugary low-fat vanilla latte for this delicious and frothy breakfast beverage. By loading up on healthy fats in the morning, you are giving your brain an amazing fuel source that will keep you satiated well into the afternoon. If you don't do dairy, use coconut oil instead of the butter or ghee.

Place all the ingredients in a blender, and process until smooth.

PER SERVING

Macronutrients: Fat 92%; Protein 4%; Carbs 4%

Calories: 584; Total Fat: 60g; Protein: 5g; Total Carbs: 6g; Fiber: 3g; Net Carbs: 3g

GREEN TEA LATTE

YIELD: *1 serving (16.5 ounces)*

1½ cups brewed green tea or brewed matcha tea

½ cup unsweetened full-fat coconut milk

1 tablespoon MCT oil

Green tea and matcha tea both come from the same plant but are grown differently. Matcha tea bushes are shaded prior to harvest to stimulate increased chlorophyll levels. Both teas are great for energy and are known in Japan as the "antiaging beverage," so this latte is perfect for the non-coffee-drinkers out there or for anyone looking to mix up their morning routine.

Place all the ingredients in a blender, and process until smooth.

PER SERVING
Macronutrients: Fat 92%; Protein 3%; Carbs 5%
Calories: 342; Total Fat: 35g; Protein: 2g; Total Carbs: 5g; Fiber: 2g; Net Carbs: 3g

KETO HOT CHOCOLATE

YIELD: 1 serving (8.5 ounces)

1 cup unsweetened full-fat coconut milk

1 teaspoon cacao powder

½ teaspoon stevia *or* 4 drops liquid stevia extract

I live in New York City, and there is no better time of year than the holiday season. The city is full of sparkling lights, festive storefronts, and holiday markets. I love making a double batch of this hot chocolate to keep my husband and me warm as we head outside to experience all the holiday fun.

1. Combine the coconut milk, cacao powder, and stevia in a small saucepan over medium heat.

2. Stir continuously until the mixture is heated through and just starting to bubble.

3. Pour the cocoa into a travel mug, and head outside!

PER SERVING

Macronutrients: Fat 86%; Protein 4%; Carbs 10%
Calories: 482; Total Fat: 46g; Protein: 5g; Total Carbs: 12g; Fiber: 6g; Net Carbs: 6g

KETO LEMONADE OR LIMEADE

YIELD: *8 servings (1 cup per serving)*

8 cups water

½ cup freshly squeezed
lemon or lime juice

1 teaspoon stevia
or 8 drops liquid
stevia extract

This drink is incredibly refreshing on a hot summer day. I'll make a big batch at the beginning of the week and store it in a pitcher in the refrigerator. Use freshly squeezed juice for the best flavor.

1. Pour the water into a pitcher.

2. Add the lemon or lime juice and stevia.

3. Stir well until combined.

4. Store in the refrigerator, and enjoy throughout the week.

CKL TIP: For extra electrolytes, add a pinch of pink Himalayan salt.

PER SERVING
Macronutrients: Fat 0%; Protein 0%; Carbs 100%
Calories: 6; Total Fat: 0g; Protein: 0g; Total Carbs: 2g; Fiber: 0g; Net Carbs: 2g

PREP TIME: 5 minutes
COOK TIME: 18 to 72 hours

BONE BROTH

YIELD: *12 to 16 servings (1 to 1¼ cups per serving)*

2 pounds beef or chicken bones, or a combination

2 carrots, coarsely chopped

2 celery stalks, coarsely chopped

1 white onion, coarsely chopped

2 garlic cloves, halved

1 tablespoon pink Himalayan salt

2 tablespoons apple cider vinegar

The benefits of bone broth are incredible. I used bone broth to treat my leaky gut when I was battling ulcerative colitis, and I still drink it on a regular basis. Freeze any bones from the meat you cook until you have enough for the recipe. You can also place an order for bones with your butcher.

1. Place the bones, carrots, celery, onion, and garlic in a slow cooker.

2. Add enough water to cover the bones and vegetables entirely.

3. Add the salt and the apple cider vinegar.

4. Set the slow cooker on low, and cook for 18 to 72 hours.

5. Line a colander with cheesecloth, and set it over a large bowl. Strain the broth through the prepared colander. Discard the bones. Let the broth cool to room temperature.

6. A good broth will usually develop a layer of fat on the top when it cools. Remove the fat with a spoon, and discard.

7. Store the broth in large mason jars in the refrigerator for up to a week, or freeze for up to 6 months.

CKL TIP: Save your vegetable scraps and leftover bones in a large zip-top bag in the freezer to use in your bone broth.

PER SERVING
Macronutrients: Fat 64%; Protein 23%; Carbs 13%
Calories: 70; Total Fat: 5g; Protein: 4g; Total Carbs: 1g; Fiber: 0g; Net Carbs: 1g

LIME MARGARITA

YIELD: *1 serving (8 ounces)*

2 tablespoons coarse sea salt

Lime wedge

Ice cubes

2 ounces 100% agave tequila

6 ounces sparkling water or club soda

1 tablespoon freshly squeezed lime juice

Stevia

My friends know that I love a good tequila cocktail, so of course I had to create a keto-friendly margarita. Enjoy!

1. Spread the salt out in an even layer on a small plate.

2. Rub a lime wedge around the rim of a glass, and dip it into the plate of salt to create a salt rim.

3. Fill the glass with ice cubes.

4. Pour the tequila, sparkling water, lime juice, and stevia to taste into a cocktail shaker. Shake well, pour into the glass, and enjoy.

PER SERVING
Macronutrients: Fat 0%; Protein 0%; Carbs 100%
Calories: 145; Total Fat: 0g; Protein: 0g; Total Carbs: 1g; Fiber: 0g; Net Carbs: 1g

KETO MOJITO

YIELD: *1 serving (8 ounces)*

10 fresh mint leaves,
plus more for garnish

Ice cubes

2 ounces rum

6 ounces sparkling water
or club soda

1 tablespoon freshly
squeezed lime juice

Stevia

Fresh mint is what makes mojitos so distinctive and refreshing. Drinking them reminds me of good times poolside on an extended tropical vacation. If you can't get away, at least you can drink this.

1. Put the mint leaves in a glass and muddle them with the handle of a wooden spoon or a muddler, if you have one.

2. Fill the glass with ice cubes.

3. Pour the rum, sparkling water, lime juice, and stevia to taste into a cocktail shaker. Shake well, and pour into the glass.

4. Garnish with more mint.

PER SERVING
Macronutrients: Fat 0%; Protein 0%; Carbs 100%
Calories: 139; Total Fat: 0g; Protein: 0g; Total Carbs: 2g; Fiber: 1g; Net Carbs: 1g

VODKA LEMONADE

YIELD: *1 serving (8 ounces)*

Ice cubes

2 ounces vodka

6 ounces Keto Lemonade
(page 161)

4 frozen strawberries
(optional)

This simple cocktail combines vodka with lemonade for a tart and refreshing adult beverage. Throw in a few frozen strawberries to add some color and sweetness to your glass.

1. Fill a tall glass with ice cubes.

2. Pour the vodka and Keto Lemonade into a cocktail shaker. Shake well, and pour into the glass.

3. Add in a few frozen strawberries (if using), and serve.

PER SERVING
Macronutrients: Fat 0%; Protein 0%; Carbs 100%
Calories: 137; Total Fat: 0g; Protein: 0g; Total Carbs: 2g; Fiber: 0g; Net Carbs: 2g

WHITE WINE SPRITZER

YIELD: *1 serving (8 ounces)*

Ice cubes

6 ounces chilled dry
white wine

2 ounces sparkling water
or club soda

Slice of lemon or lime,
for garnish

I have become a huge fan of wine spritzers. They are cool, crisp, and classy. Opt for low-carb white wines such as pinot grigio, chardonnay, or sauvignon blanc when making this drink.

1. Fill a wine glass with ice cubes.

2. Pour the wine into the glass, followed by the sparkling water.

3. Garnish with the lemon or lime slice, and serve.

PER SERVING
Macronutrients: Fat 0%; Protein 0%; Carbs 100%
Calories: 141; Total Fat: 0g; Protein: 0g; Total Carbs: 5g; Fiber: 0g; Net Carbs: 5g

BERRY SANGRIA

YIELD: *1 serving (8 ounces)*

Ice cubes

6 ounces chilled dry
   red wine

2 ounces sugar-free
   berry-flavored
   sparkling water

¼ cup frozen mixed
   berries (blueberries,
   raspberries,
   blackberries)

This is an all-around crowd-pleaser that will work nicely at your next party or holiday gathering. Calculate how many servings you need, and adjust the recipe accordingly. Pour it into a large pitcher or punch bowl.

1. Fill a wine glass with ice cubes.

2. Pour the wine into the glass, followed by the berry-flavored sparkling water.

3. Toss in the berries, and serve.

PER SERVING
Macronutrients: Fat 0%; Protein 0%; Carbs 100%
Calories: 163; Total Fat: 0g; Protein: 0g; Total Carbs: 8g; Fiber: 1g; Net Carbs: 7g

PECAN CLUSTERS

YIELD: *6 servings (1 cluster per serving)*

3 tablespoons
grass-fed butter

¼ cup heavy cream

½ teaspoon stevia
or 4 drops liquid
stevia extract

½ teaspoon vanilla extract

¼ teaspoon pink
Himalayan salt

1 cup pecans, chopped

Caramel and nuts really are an amazing pairing, which is what inspired me to create these Pecan Clusters. They are rich, creamy, and delicious. Store them in the refrigerator to ensure that they stay solid.

1. Line a baking sheet with parchment paper.

2. In a small saucepan, melt the butter over medium heat until it turns golden, 2 to 3 minutes, stirring frequently to avoid burning.

3. Whisk in the heavy cream until combined.

4. Turn the heat to low and, whisking quickly, add the stevia, vanilla, and salt, making sure to break up any lumps.

5. Continue to whisk occasionally for 5 minutes as the mixture begins to thicken. It should have a consistency similar to caramel and will darken slightly in color.

6. Remove from the heat, and mix in the chopped pecans.

7. Drop teaspoonfuls of the caramel-pecan mixture onto the prepared baking sheet.

8. Place the baking sheet in the freezer for 10 minutes.

9. Transfer the clusters to a sealed container, and store in the refrigerator.

PER SERVING
Macronutrients: Fat 94%; Protein 3%; Carbs 3%
Calories: 125; Total Fat: 13g; Protein: 1g; Total Carbs: 1g; Fiber: 1g; Net Carbs: 0g

MACADAMIA LIME BITES

YIELD: *16 servings (1 bite per serving)*

⅓ cup coconut oil, melted, plus more for greasing

1 cup macadamia nuts, raw or dry roasted

¼ cup unsweetened full-fat coconut milk

3 tablespoons freshly squeezed lime juice

1 teaspoon lime zest

1 teaspoon vanilla extract

½ teaspoon stevia
or 4 drops liquid stevia extract

1 tablespoon coconut flour

This recipe was inspired by my love of Key lime pie. Using buttery macadamia nuts as the base, these lime bites are a decadent treat. If you have access to Key lime juice, definitely use it. Otherwise, regular lime juice does the trick.

1. Grease an ice cube tray with coconut oil.

2. Combine all the ingredients in a food processor, and process until well combined. The mixture should have the consistency of a thick and creamy nut butter.

3. Transfer the mixture to the ice cube tray, and place it in the freezer for at least 30 minutes or until the cubes are solid and firm.

4. Transfer the bites to a sealed container, and store them in the freezer.

PER SERVING
Macronutrients: Fat 89%; Protein 3%; Carbs 8%
Calories: 111; Total Fat: 11g; Protein: 1g; Total Carbs: 2g; Fiber: 1g; Net Carbs: 1g

COCONUT COOKIES

YIELD: *6 servings (1 cookie per serving)*

2 tablespoons
grass-fed butter

⅔ cup almond butter

1 tablespoon cacao powder
(optional)

1 teaspoon stevia
or 8 drops liquid
stevia extract

1 cup unsweetened
shredded coconut

I am crazy about coconut! These cookies require no baking and can be made with or without cacao, depending on your preference. Either way, they have a craveable coconutty taste I cannot resist.

1. Line a baking sheet with parchment paper.

2. In a small saucepan, melt the butter over medium heat.

3. Pour the melted butter into a medium bowl, stir in the almond butter, and mix until smooth.

4. Mix in the cocoa powder (if using).

5. Add the stevia and coconut, and mix thoroughly.

6. Drop 2-inch spoonfuls of the mixture onto the prepared baking sheet.

7. Freeze for at least 10 minutes or until they are completely solidified.

8. Transfer the cookies to a sealed container, and store in the refrigerator.

PER SERVING
Macronutrients: Fat 82%; Protein 6%; Carbs 12%
Calories: 315; Total Fat: 31g; Protein: 5g; Total Carbs: 10g; Fiber: 4g; Net Carbs: 6g

CHOCO-AVO PUDDING

YIELD: *1 serving*

1 avocado, pitted and peeled, then chilled for at least 2 hours

⅓ cup unsweetened full-fat coconut milk

2 tablespoons cacao powder

½ teaspoon stevia *or* 4 drops liquid stevia extract

½ teaspoon vanilla extract

¼ teaspoon pink Himalayan salt

Avocado makes everything richer and smoother, and that includes pudding. When you make this, you'll see that it rivals any store-bought brand when it comes to taste and texture. Top this pudding with some shredded coconut flakes or cacao nibs for a satisfying keto dessert. Don't forget to chill the avocado in advance.

1. Place all the ingredients in a blender or food processor.
2. Blend thoroughly until smooth.
3. Eat right away, or refrigerate it for at least 1 hour for a more mousse-like consistency.

CKL TIP: Halve, pit, and peel ripe avocados, and store them in the freezer in a sealed container for use in puddings and smoothies.

PER SERVING
Macronutrients: Fat 77%; Protein 5%; Carbs 18%
Calories: 414; Total Fat: 38g; Protein: 6g; Total Carbs: 20g; Fiber: 11g; Net Carbs: 9g

CHOCOLATE FUDGE

YIELD: *12 servings (1 square per serving)*

1 cup coconut oil

¼ cup cacao powder

½ teaspoon stevia
  or 4 drops liquid
  stevia extract

1 teaspoon vanilla extract

¼ cup almond butter

¼ teaspoon pink
  Himalayan salt

Ready to have the best fudge ever? Say hello to this recipe that is by far my most popular keto confection. I always have this fudge on hand in my freezer for when I am in the mood for something sweet and salty.

1. Line a 5-by-5-inch square dish with parchment paper overhanging the sides.

2. In a small saucepan, melt the coconut oil over low heat.

3. Add the cacao and stevia, and stir until completely smooth.

4. Remove from the heat, and stir in the vanilla.

5. Taste and add additional stevia if you prefer more sweetness.

6. Pour the mixture into the prepared dish.

7. Swirl the almond butter over the top, and sprinkle with the salt.

8. Freeze for 30 minutes or until solid and firm.

9. Using the parchment paper as handles, carefully transfer the fudge to a cutting board.

10. Cut the fudge into squares, and store them in a sealed container in the freezer.

PER SERVING

Macronutrients: Fat 88%; Protein 4%; Carbs 8%
Calories: 235; Total Fat: 23g; Protein: 2g; Total Carbs: 5g; Fiber: 2g; Net Carbs: 3g

FINAL THOUGHTS

Friends and future CKL pros,

I am so honored that you have taken the time to read this book, soak up all the information in it, and are open to the idea of living a Clean Keto Lifestyle!

Often when starting the keto journey, my clients ask me how long they need to stay keto, and I tell them "ideally—for life!" The truth is that if you go back to mainly eating carbs and sugars, your body will jump right back onto the "glu-coaster," and all the amazing benefits you've experienced from being in ketosis will go away.

And yet, now that you've completed my program, you know the truth about why this statement isn't as scary as it initially seems: after the first month of being keto, my clients almost always report that they have *no desire* to go back to their old way of living. In fact, they feel so good and so energized that the thought of doing anything but keto doesn't seem appealing. I hope that at this point in your journey, you are feeling that way, too. I also hope that my advice, tips, and meal plans have given you all the tools you need to take action, stay motivated, and make this a long-term and sustainable lifestyle.

It *is* possible. I know because I am living proof of how powerful and life-changing fueling your body with the proper foods can be.

Does this mean that you can never have a piece of bread again and not allow one ounce of sugar to enter your body forever? No way. After about 14–30 days of being keto, your body will become "keto-adapted," which means it can effortlessly run on its own fat stores for energy and is very good at getting back into ketosis if you ingest too many carbs at a meal. So there will always be a time and place for a few indulgences once in a while, but for the most part you should be eating the CKL way on a regular basis.

I made this book as comprehensive as possible to ensure that you have everything that you need to succeed. But please feel free to reach out to me if you have any further questions, comments, or want to share your success story! You can get in touch with me via my website (CleanKetoLifestyle.com) or my social media channels (@CleanKetoLifestyle).

I am so excited for you to transform your life, and I hope one day we have the chance to meet and share stories!

xoxo

Karissa

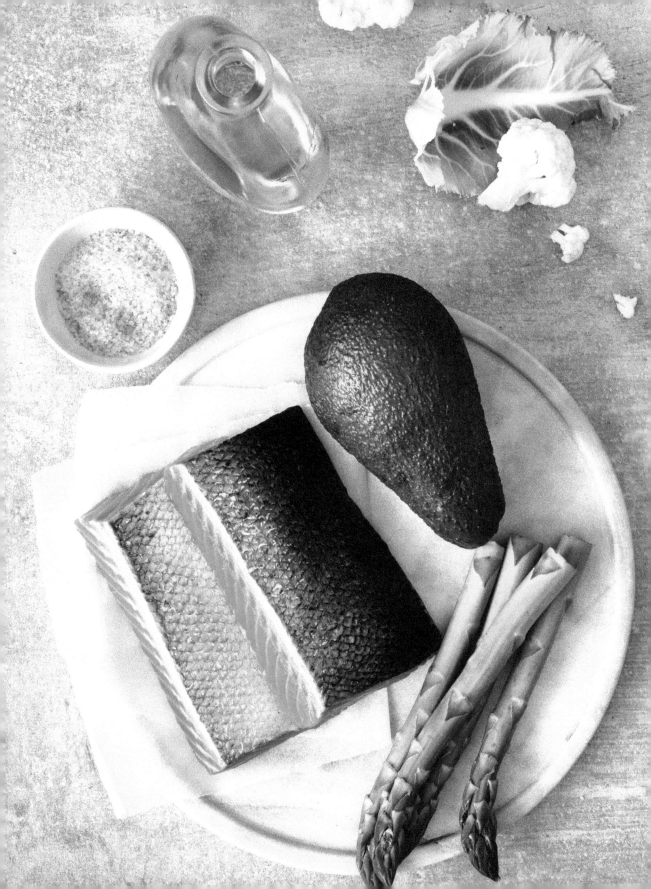

MEASUREMENT CONVERSIONS

VOLUME EQUIVALENTS (LIQUID)

US Standard	US Standard (ounces)	Metric (approximate)
2 tablespoons	1 fl. oz.	30 mL
¼ cup	2 fl. oz.	60 mL
½ cup	4 fl. oz.	120 mL
1 cup	8 fl. oz.	240 mL
1½ cups	12 fl. oz.	355 mL
2 cups or 1 pint	16 fl. oz.	475 mL
4 cups or 1 quart	32 fl. oz.	1 L
1 gallon	128 fl. oz.	4 L

OVEN TEMPERATURES

Fahrenheit (F)	Celsius (C) (approximate)
250°F	120°C
300°F	150°C
325°F	165°C
350°F	180°C
375°F	190°C
400°F	200°C
425°F	220°C
450°F	230°C

VOLUME EQUIVALENTS (DRY)

US Standard	Metric (approximate)
⅛ teaspoon	0.5 mL
¼ teaspoon	1 mL
½ teaspoon	2 mL
¾ teaspoon	4 mL
1 teaspoon	5 mL
1 tablespoon	15 mL
¼ cup	59 mL
⅓ cup	79 mL
½ cup	118 mL
⅔ cup	156 mL
¾ cup	177 mL
1 cup	235 mL
2 cups or 1 pint	475 mL
3 cups	700 mL
4 cups or 1 quart	1 L

WEIGHT EQUIVALENTS

US Standard	Metric (approximate)
½ ounce	15 g
1 ounce	30 g
2 ounces	60 g
4 ounces	115 g
8 ounces	225 g
12 ounces	340 g
16 ounces or 1 pound	455 g

KETO RESOURCES

Looking for even more keto inspiration? Here are my go-to resources on all things keto!

CleanKetoLifestyle.com: Head over to the official CKL website to access free resources, get recipe inspiration, and connect with me.

Bacon and Butter, by Celby Richoux: I mean, could there be a better title for a keto cookbook? This book has 150 keto-friendly recipes designed to keep your taste buds very happy.

The Easy 5-Ingredient Ketogenic Diet Cookbook, by Jen Fisch: Simplify your life with this wonderful cookbook that will have you eating tasty keto dishes—using five ingredients or less!

The Big Book of Ketogenic Diet Cooking, by Jen Fisch: This book is filled with 200 delicious keto recipes to add to your rotation and ensure you have plenty of variety in your diet.

The Keto Instant Pot Cookbook, by Urvashi Pitre: As an electric slow cooker and pressure cooker combined, the Instant Pot will soon be your best friend in the kitchen. You can whip up soups, ribs, and even a batch of bone broth with little effort and in a fraction of the time it would ordinarily take you. This book will show you how and what to cook to make amazing keto dishes. And of course, the recipes are delicious.

REFERENCES

Barañano, Kristen W., MD, PhD and Adam L. Hartman, MD. "The Ketogenic Diet: Uses in Epilepsy and Other Neurologic Illnesses." *Current Treatment Options in Neurology* 10, no. 6 (November 2008): 410–19. Accessed August 28, 2018. https://www.ncbi.nlm.nih.gov/pmc/articles/PMC2898565/.

Hertz, Leif, Ye Chen, and Helle S. Waagepetersen. "Effects of Ketone Bodies in Alzheimer's Disease in Relation to Neural Hypometabolism, β-amyloid Toxicity, and Astrocyte Function." *Journal of Neurochemistry* 134, no. 1 (July 2015): 7–20. doi: 10.1111/jnc.13107. Accessed August 28, 2018. https://www.ncbi.nlm.nih.gov/pubmed/25832906.

Maciej Gasior, Michael A. Rogawski, and Adam L. Hartmana. "Neuroprotective and Disease-Modifying Effects of the Ketogenic Diet." *Behavioural Pharmacology* 17, no. 5–6 (September 2006): 431–39. Accessed August 28, 2018. https://www.ncbi.nlm.nih.gov/pmc/articles/PMC2367001/.

Storoni, Mithu and Gordon T. Plant. "The Therapeutic Potential of the Ketogenic Diet in Treating Progressive Multiple Sclerosis." Multiple Sclerosis International (2015): 681289. doi: 10.1155/2015/681289. Accessed August 28, 2018. https://www.ncbi.nlm.nih.gov/pmc/articles/PMC4709725/.

Weber, Daniela D., Sepideh Aminazdeh-Gohari, and Barbara Kofler. *Open-Access Impact Journal on Aging* 10, no. 2 (February 2018). doi:10.18632/aging.101382. Accessed August 28, 2018. https://www.ncbi.nlm.nih.gov/pmc/articles/PMC5842847/.

White, Hayden and Balasubramanian Venkatesh. "Clinical Review: Ketones and Brain Injury." *Critical Care* 15, no. 2 (April 6, 2011): 219. doi:10.1186/cc10020. Accessed August 28, 2018. https://onlinelibrary.wiley.com/doi/full/10.1111/jnc.13107.

RECIPE INDEX

INDEX

Sides
    Asian Spiced
        Cucumbers, 116
    Cauliflower Mash, 109
    Creamed Spinach, 115
    Crispy Brussels Sprouts, 110
    Garlicky Kale, 114
    Mexican Cauliflower
        Rice, 111
    Roasted Broccoli, 108
    Roasted Mushrooms, 112
    Sautéed Summer
        Squash, 113
    Southern Green Beans, 117
Smoothies and shakes
    Berry Cheesecake
        Smoothie, 104
    Chocolate Protein
        Shake, 105
    Green Smoothie, 103
Snacks, 38
Social gatherings, 72, 74
Soups and stews
    Chicken Tortilla Soup, 128
    Slow Cooker Keto Chili, 129
Spinach
    Chocolate Protein
        Shake, 105
    Creamed Spinach, 115
    Green Smoothie, 103
    Italian Omelet, 100
    Italian Zoodles, 149

    Prosciutto Egg Cups, 98
    Spinach Bacon Salad, 125
    Turkey Egg Scramble, 96
    Zesty Chicken Tender
        Salad, 124
Squash. *See also* Zucchini
    Sautéed Summer
        Squash, 113
Staple ingredients, 25–
    27, 36–37
Substitutions, 35
Supplements, 55
Support systems, 77

T

Tea
    Green Tea Latte, 159
Testing ketones, 55
Tomatoes
    Balsamic Chicken, 140
    Basil Chicken Zucchini
        "Pasta," 139
    Chef Salad, 122
    Chicken Tortilla Soup, 128
    Chopped Salad, 123
    Italian Omelet, 100
    Italian Tuna Salad, 121
    Shrimp & Avocado
        Salad, 120
    Steak Salad, 127
Triglycerides, 5, 17

Turkey
    Turkey Egg Scramble, 96
    Turkey Meatballs, 141
    Turkey Taco Bowl, 138

V

Vegans, 38–39
Vegetables, 39. *See also specific*
Vegetarians, 38–39

W

Water, 32, 60
Weight loss, 7
Wine
    Berry Sangria, 167
    White Wine Spritzer, 166

Z

Zucchini
    Basil Chicken Zucchini
        "Pasta," 139
    Italian Zoodles, 149
    Mini Burger Sliders, 147
    Roasted Shrimp &
        Veggies, 132
    Sautéed Summer
        Squash, 113

ACKNOWLEDGMENTS

First and foremost, thank you to all my clients who inspire me every single day. Thank you for trusting me, my programs, and my method. Your unwavering passion, dedication, and determination to put your health first and make positive changes in your life is what drives me to do what I do. There is nothing better than seeing your incredible transformations and waking up every morning to texts/e-mails/pictures detailing your successes. I am forever grateful for each and every one of you.

To my parents and three younger siblings who have given me so much support throughout my life and who provide me with unconditional love every single day: all of you in your own way gave me invaluable help on this book.

And finally, to my husband, for his constant patience, support, and encouragement. His endless belief in me and my dreams are the reason this book exists. He is simply the best, and I love him more than avocado!

ABOUT THE AUTHOR

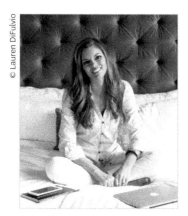

As a global health coach trained by the Institute for Integrative Nutrition, **Karissa Long** successfully guides her clients through the process of changing their relationships with food, creating healthy habits (even if they have busy schedules), and achieving optimal health using the ketogenic diet. Karissa's mission is to help every person feel empowered to change their health for the better through a Clean Keto Lifestyle. This means doing the ketogenic diet the right way: free of processed foods and artificial ingredients, and full of real whole foods. Karissa is also the founder and CEO of Clean Keto Lifestyle. Her proprietary keto programs are designed to give everyone the tools they need to achieve optimum vitality and live their best lives through the following principles: nourish, heal, and thrive. Karissa has spent over a decade transforming and fine-tuning her own health, and researching how what we put in our bodies and how we live our lives impacts our overall well-being. She went from a fast-food-eating, soda-pop-drinking sugar addict to a clean-eating, fat-burning machine! She found the ketogenic diet during her personal struggles with a debilitating autoimmune disease, and it completely transformed her life.

CleanKetoLifestyle.com
Follow Karissa on 🐦 f 📌 📷 @CleanKetoLifestyle

CPSIA information can be obtained
at www.ICGtesting.com
Printed in the USA
BVHW051906161118
533078BV00001B/1/P